P9-DNA-203

YOUR CHILD'S MOTOR DEVELOPMENT STORY

Understanding and Enhancing Development from Birth to Their First Sport

By
Jill Howlett Mays, MS, OTR/L

YOUR CHILD'S MOTOR DEVELOPMENT STORY:

Understanding and Enhancing Development from Birth to Their First Sport

All marketing and publishing rights guaranteed to and reserved by:

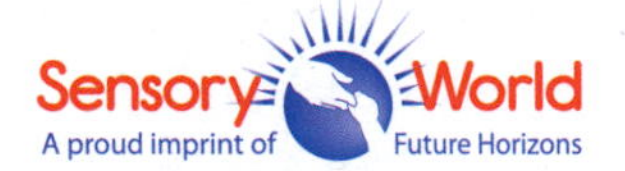

1010 N Davis Dr
Arlington, TX 76012
(877) 775-8968
(682) 558-8941
(682) 558-8945 (fax)
E-mail: *info@sensoryworld.com*
www.sensoryworld.com

©2011 Jill Howlett Mays
Photography by Eileen Counihan
Interior design by Cindy Williams
Cover design by John Yacio, III

All rights reserved.
Printed in Canada.

No part of this product may be reproduced in any manner whatsoever without written permission of Future Horizons, Inc, except in the case of brief quotations embodied in reviews.

ISBN no. 9781935567325

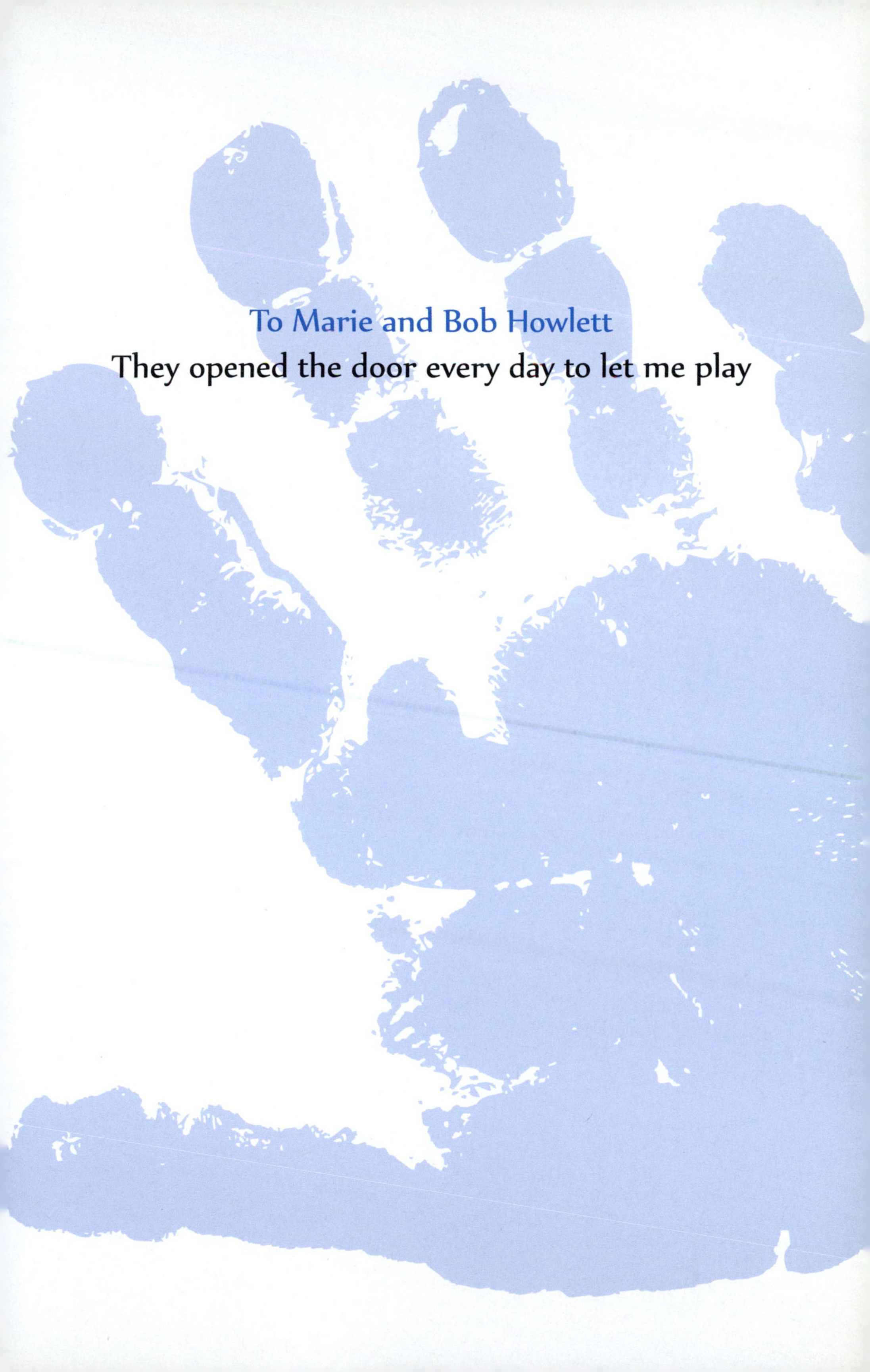

To Marie and Bob Howlett

They opened the door every day to let me play

Acknowledgments

First, I'd like to thank Kate Mays for her prepublishing efforts and advice. It's a difficult task to critique someone's work, especially when it's your mother's. Ben Mays patiently showed me how to expand my limited computer skills and has been my ongoing "tech" support.

There were many who helped nudge this book forward. Betsy McKenna and Maureen Murphy, both leaders in childhood education, critiqued numerous drafts. Dr Jules Spotts, child psychologist; Ailene Tisser, physical therapist; and Nancy Wergeles, family therapist, shared their professional viewpoints. Carol Mack, award-winning playwright and author, took the time to review the text and helped make each chapter "pop." Authors Jeff Wilser and Amy Kalafa pushed me to find a publisher. Thuy Tranthi, business executive and mother of beautiful Ariel, lent her sharp marketing eye and found the information on "overscheduling" a useful personal guide as she negotiated the preschool years. Carrie Gitzes, Lili Monge, Beth O'Brien, Erin Golden, and Kathleen Tuttle all provided invaluable feedback.

Special thanks to the mothers who brought their children to the photo shoot: Annabelle Alt, Calma Lewis, Keerthi Kongettira, and Suzanne Cartell. They are gifted educators in their own right and bring their understanding of development to their own children. Thanks especially to Elisa, Wayne, Vedha, Aanya, Harrison, and Bobby for illustrating what healthy, normal development and play look like. Eileen Counihan, photographer extraordinaire, you captured this beautifully. Thanks also to Lili Monge, Natalie Hodges, and Leslie Brown for allowing me to use personal photos of their wonderful boys!

I'd like to thank Marjorie Becker-Lewin, who enhanced my knowledge of sensory integration and how to put Jean Ayres's theories into practice. Stanley Greenspan was the first child psychiatrist to recognize and broadcast the importance of sensorimotor development and play for the social, emotional, and physical well-being of all children. Drs Ayres and Greenspan have left this world, but their legacy will continue to change the lives of countless children and their families.

Pat Oakes introduced me to Carol Stock Kranowitz, who told the world what sensory integration is about in her "Out-of-Sync" books.

Carol introduced me to Jennifer Gilpin of Future Horizons, who had the vision to see that motor development is important not just to "special-needs populations," but to normally developing children, as well. Cindy Williams and Heather Babiar helped bring the book to press. Thank you, all!

Finally, I'd like to thank my son, Christopher, for sharing his son, Bobby, for all of the photo shoots and videos. And to Eric, because you keep everything in our lives moving forward.

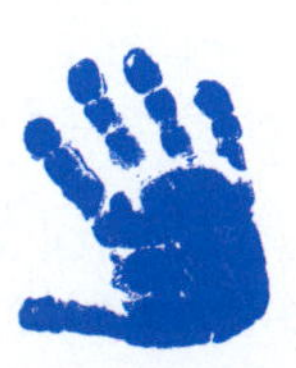

Table of Contents

Introduction

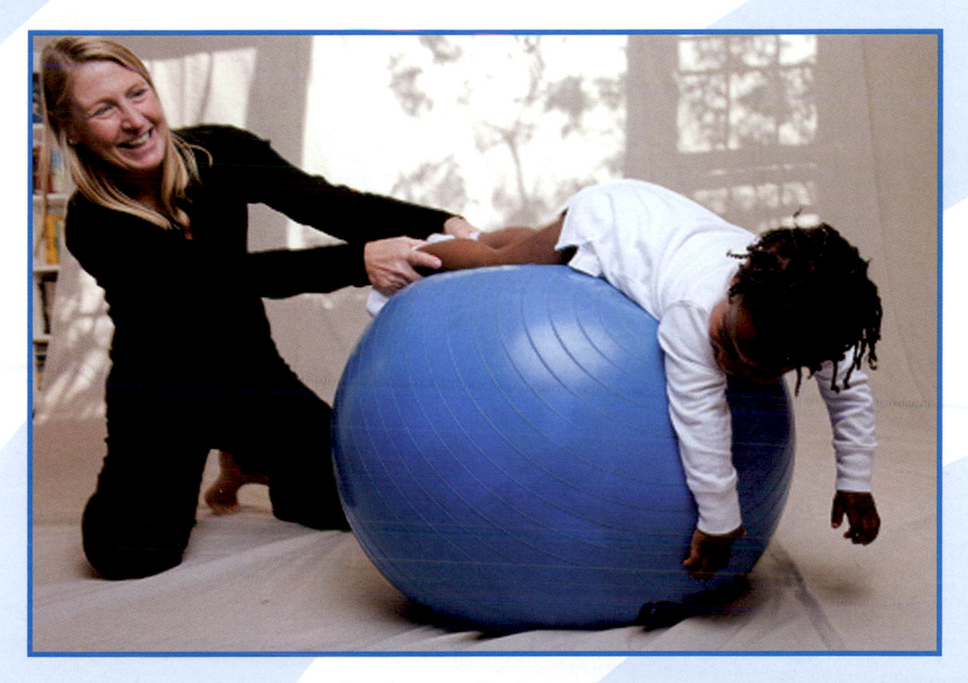

Figure 1. Jill plays with her friend Wayne.

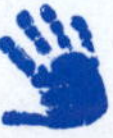

"I can't do it!" Timmy sobbed. He slumped over the scooter board. "I can't do any more!"

Flying across the room like Superman on a scooter normally delights children, but this activity overwhelmed Timmy. He lacked the strength and coordination to kick off of the wall successfully.

Timmy's pediatrician referred him to me for occupational therapy. A range of problems had been identified at school. He avoided all tabletop activities and ran away during circle time, especially when singing and dancing were involved. He frequently hid under the table. At home, Timmy cried and lost his temper on a regular basis. His dad spent time playing catch with him, but after Timmy tossed the ball one or two times, he crumbled. It was not a positive bonding experience.

A "sensorimotor assessment" revealed that Timmy's body was not strong and that he became confused about how to move his body when trying new activities. Over a year of therapy, he became considerably stronger, and his stamina improved. Timmy gained confidence in his body movements. With increased body awareness, he took more risks and even began to challenge himself. Baseball sessions with Dad became enjoyable as his eye-hand coordination improved. Most importantly, Timmy no longer fell apart each time he was confronted with a new physical challenge. The tantrums he had at school and at home resulted from the fatigue caused by the many stresses he experienced throughout the day.

By the time Timmy reached first grade, he managed his classroom activities well. He had become a much calmer and happier child. Ironically, gross-motor activities (activities involving large muscle groups and whole-body movements) became his preferred choice during playtime. Two years later, Timmy's mother reported that he was ranked number three out of a field of hundreds in his town's Triple-A Little League tryouts.

I have worked with children for more than 30 years. My practice has focused on helping children develop confidence as they learn to move around and be comfortable as they cope with their ever-expanding environment. A child's world begins in the nursery. Some infants struggle soon after birth. All the stimulation surrounding them can be overwhelming: sounds, lights, touch sensations, and movements. It can be

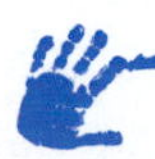

difficult for these babies to be soothed. The demands can increase as a child moves into the daycare setting. New faces and sounds, new toys to play with, other children close by—all this requires more sophisticated neurological organization of a child's sensorimotor system. Many children make the leap with ease. For others, it is an uphill climb.

Thirty years ago, when parents expressed concern regarding their child's motor ability, pediatricians would frequently say, "Not to worry…he'll grow out of it." Since that time, child studies have shown that some children exhibit differences in motor development that they do not "grow out of." Indeed, recent studies in brain development have shown subtle differences in the brain chemistry of some children that correspond with differences in their motor behavior. These differences affect not only physical coordination, but also attention, concentration, and emotion.

Happily, conventional wisdom now recognizes the pivotal role early intervention has in helping children acquire the skills they need in all areas of development. For example, when a child is "language delayed," early speech therapy can jump-start communication skills. As language skills improve, learning to read comes more easily. Similarly, when children struggle to learn basic motor skills, receiving early support makes it easier for them to gain confidence not only on the playground and in the gym, but also in the classroom. Awareness and caring intervention from birth are very powerful and can prevent later problems.

In preschool, a child is expected to play with toys and games according to rules. "Performance" begins to matter in a new way. The child who happily looked at picture books for hours is suddenly asked to climb on an outdoor structure, play "Hokey Pokey," and touch play dough, shaving cream, and other gooey substances. The very physical child, who would spend hours climbing the playground structure, is now asked to sit quietly for story time and draw pictures at a table.

As a child enters kindergarten, there are even greater demands to be met. Once elementary school begins, the child is expected to quickly master writing and reading. To accomplish these tasks, *underlying physical skills must be in place*. These include the basic ability to sit at a desk or in a circle, to sit comfortably next to another student, and to know

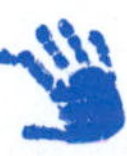

how to walk with a group (usually single file). When math time comes, it is assumed that the child can comfortably manipulate toys like Unifix cubes and be able to cut out shapes. At this point, for children who do not possess skills the rest of us take for granted, a big struggle ensues in the classroom. Frequently, these children are referred to me.

Many of the children I work with have not developed the core strength necessary to sit for extended periods at their desks or on the floor. They might slouch, or, if allowed, might roll around. Sometimes these students unwittingly create a disturbance in the classroom. In one very progressive school where I worked, a child preferred to stand on his head! This actually helped him pay attention. Many children have not developed the strength or hand-coordination necessary to manipulate all of the items they're required to use at school: pencils, scissors, tape dispensers, sharpeners, cards, and paper clips. For some, even putting papers into folders can be a struggle. These children end up with backpacks filled with a mess of crushed and crumpled paper and a desk overflowing with papers, pencils, and crayons.

The children in my caseload range from highly gifted children with subtle motor or perceptual difficulties to children struggling with autism and other neurological impairments. Some are learning to cope with attention-deficit disorder or attention-deficit/hyperactivity disorder. Others have experienced delays in certain aspects of their physical or neurological development. The children are referred for a variety of reasons: troubles with handwriting, fine-motor difficulties, clumsiness, and/or hypersensitivities to touch.

What underlies these difficulties varies case by case. *Many problems point back to early development and difficulties with sensorimotor processing*. It may involve weak trunk strength, difficulty coordinating the two sides of the body, problems with executing a series of movements, a tendency to become overwhelmed by sensations, or lack of confidence in how the body moves. In most of these cases, *early emphasis on sensorimotor development would prevent or limit the difficulties seen later.*

When I review these issues during parent conferences, teacher workshops, and lectures, an "Aha" moment usually occurs. As I describe how the pieces of a child's motor

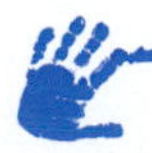

development are put together—the interplay of the senses and behavior—a picture of the child emerges that radiates a new understanding of *why* the child might behave in certain ways. Often the necessary *bedrock* for later performance is not solid. With a shifting or weak sensorimotor base, the child's coping mechanisms are poorly adapted to environmental demands. In many cases, the child struggles from the beginning of the day until sleep finally takes over.

The need to struggle is unnecessary. The work I do during therapy is not rocket science. The time children spend with me in the clinic is essentially "playtime," in which they learn how to use their bodies more effectively. In the process of playing, they become stronger and more coordinated. Experiencing movement and different sensations in new ways leads to better processing of information. Over time, efficient body responses develop.

The Motor Story is for parents. It is intended to serve as a guide for normally developing children, as well as those who struggle with aspects of sensorimotor development. With an understanding of the basics of sensorimotor processing and motor development, parents will be able to play with their children in ways that support growth in these areas.

The most effective sensorimotor play is simple and requires no fancy equipment or programming. As a parent, you will be able to identify many activities that you already enjoy with your child but gain a new understanding of why these activities are so important. When you spend time rocking, bouncing, and moving your infant in safe and supported ways, this is helping to develop your baby's neurological system. This also helps your baby become more flexible and adaptable. Time spent crawling on the floor with a 6-month-old, a 16-month-old, and a 6-year-old will support motor development in ways that expensive toys cannot (and boutique programs can only touch on).

The chapters that follow will demonstrate how you can promote development in your child's neurological system from birth onward. With a proactive approach, later symptoms will not occur and inhibit your child's growth, causing him or her to be unhappy and frustrated. I want to share my experience to help you as a parent become more aware of the powerful effect that play can have on your child's development.

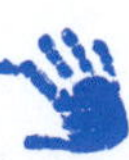

The importance of developing strong motor abilities in your child has more to do with creating a competent individual than creating an athlete. Early sensorimotor development is key to establishing many skills necessary for learning and performing in the world. *Paying attention, organizing information, and regulating emotional and behavioral responses are all influenced by how well the brain learns to process sensorimotor information.* When a child engages in a variety of play experiences that include physical activity and sensory exploration, the foundation is laid for healthy development.

Educators have understood for a long time that reading to a child from an early age is important to facilitate language comprehension and can generate a lifelong love of reading. Similarly, engaging a child in different kinds of play, varied movement experiences, and sensory exploration will help the child develop flexible and effective motor skills.

In this book, I use case studies to help you understand the concepts reviewed. While I've changed the names, these are real stories of children I have worked with over the past 30 years. The photographs are intended to illustrate healthy, normal development **(Figure 1)**. While each chapter builds upon the previous one, when reading this book, you might want to jump to the chapter most relevant to your child's particular developmental stage. Chapters 1 and 2 focus on the first year of life. Chapters 3 and 4 review the foundations of all motor skills. Chapter 5 discusses several key activities important for overall gross-motor skill development and provides suggestions on how to help your child learn these skills. Chapter 6 focuses on the athletic arena and when to make the jump to organized sports. Chapter 7 addresses motor planning, which is so important to developing successful, quality lifelong motor ability. Finally, the discussion expands to a broader context related to our values of childhood, play, and balancing the many demands currently facing our children in today's complex culture.

Parents are sincerely and highly committed to providing an enriched environment for their children to experience as they grow. Over time, however, this has translated into pressure to *buy* this "enrichment," whether it is in the form of expensive toys, elaborate home programs, or structured outside activities. Baby Einstein and "Mommy and Me" programs offer activities

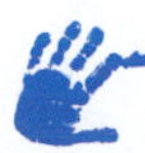

that reflect an understanding of early childhood development. The actual value of these programs is that they distill basic developmental principles and growth activities into a cookbook format to help engage a baby and child in developmentally appropriate ways. With a working understanding of the early stages of child development, parents have the tools necessary to engage their child in a thoroughly enjoyable, spontaneous, and enriching way without using expensive props.

In economically strapped times, families assess how each dollar is spent. Parents should not feel guilty about skipping a $150 infant yoga class. A top-of-the-line baby play mat, while lovely, is not necessary. Equipped with the knowledge of how to stimulate your infant and enhance his development, you will find ample supplies in your current household environment. When simple activities are coupled with actual time that you spend together engaged in play, a very happy and proficient child emerges, and the bond between you will strengthen. The ideas and activities shared within these pages will hopefully help and excite you in the rearing of your child. Understanding the benefit of many forms of play will help you hone in on the activities that will be most beneficial to your youngster's sensorimotor development. Along with exponential growth in development, the building of a loving, long-lasting relationship between you and your child will unfold.

With this book, I hope to give you a new understanding of how to proceed with your child on this amazing path of development. I have had the good fortune of sharing in the development of many extraordinary children and their wonderful families. Telling their stories and highlighting how children travel through their sensorimotor development will hopefully inspire you to begin this journey in the context of play and fun. A joyful experience awaits...

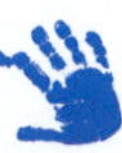

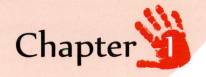

Chapter 1

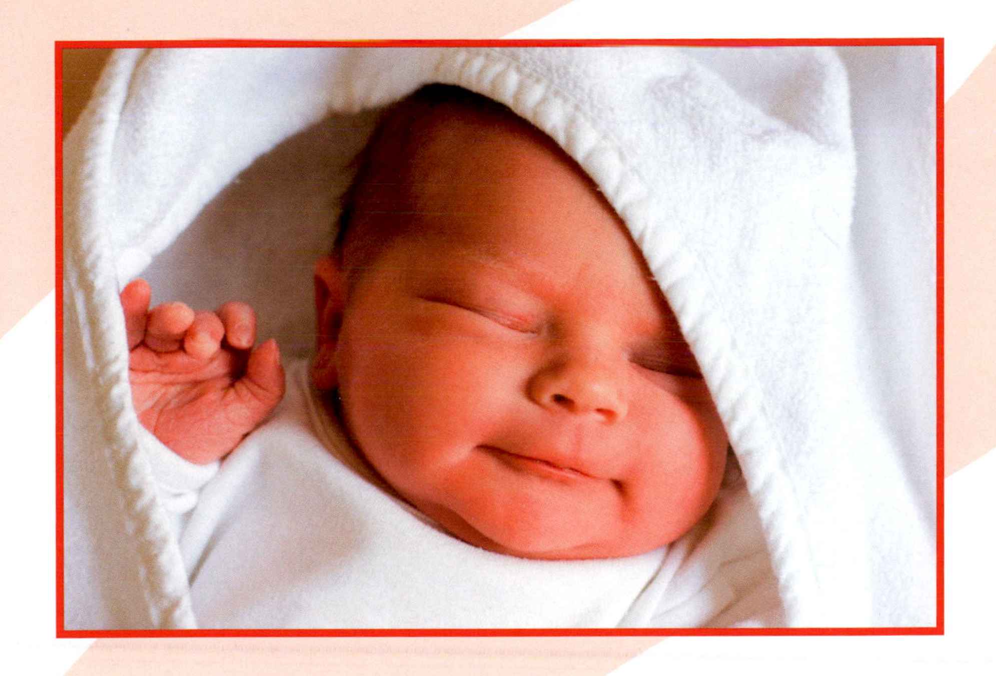

Birth and the Infant

Several children I have worked with had been adopted through the Russian orphanage system. Many of these institutions are notorious for the lack of stimulation provided to the babies. Reports indicate that they are often left in their cribs throughout the day, and interaction only occurs when they are fed. Each adopted child I have worked with has had a similar pattern. Each is referred at approximately 4 years old, after 1 year of preschool. The child is absolutely beautiful and totally engaging, and stands still for approximately a nanosecond before beginning to literally climb the walls. The reason for referral follows a similar pattern. "Very bright, engaging child, but unable to stay still in the classroom…very active but avoids tabletop activities…constantly in motion and very messy…"

While the child is isolated in that lonely crib, his or her first movements go unnoticed and unrewarded. Interesting visual and auditory stimulation is absent. The motivation to move in a goal-directed way is diminished. The opportunity to focus on an interesting toy or face, which increases early concentration and attention, does not occur. As a result, the building blocks for paying attention and developing body awareness and motor planning are missing.

The early moments of making intentional movements—swatting at a colorful mobile, reaching for a toy, and looking into a responsive caretaker's eyes—all form the basis for paying attention and performing competent movements within a child's ever-expanding world. It is critical during those early months and during a child's first year to provide opportunities for movement, cause-and-effect experiences, and generally meaningful interchanges throughout the day.

Upon assessment, children from orphanages like these share several traits. They crave all forms of sensory stimulation to the extreme. They can't move around enough, and when working with tactile materials such as paint and glue, they immerse themselves (literally!) in a very messy way. Overriding these details is a consistent inability to stay attentive to one activity for more than a few seconds. Although quite bright, each has significant visual perceptual deficits. This relates to the ability to interpret visual information in a meaningful way. For instance, they have difficulty playing "Memory" card games, "Where's

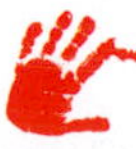

Waldo," and "I Spy" figure-ground activities (activities where you have to visually isolate objects amongst a "busy" background). Early drawings are disorganized and disconnected, even when the child has very good fine-motor control.

Treatment consists of bombarding the child with as much movement as he or she can handle. Rapid spinning on suspended swings, flying across the room on scooters, and jumping and crashing into a pile of pillows exemplify typical therapy sessions. The child covers himself in shaving cream, and family members are instructed to have him use finger-paints, make pudding drawings, and use other stimulating tactile materials every day. The child has a "tactile basket" to use whenever he needs extra sensory input, and he is allowed to use special "fidget" toys in the classroom. These "sensory diets" help to nurture a child's starving sensory system. Parents and teachers learn to understand the child's special need for extra movement and find outlets for this extraordinary reserve.

When a child has ample opportunities to move around, his ability to pay attention improves. As he gains sensorimotor experiences, spatial relationships and other visual perceptual concepts develop. Once the sensorimotor system "catches up" with corresponding brain organization, many of these adopted children exhibit artistic creativity, strong cognitive capability, and wonderful charisma.

Sasha was one such boy I worked with. He came from a Russian orphanage and was deprived of critical sensorimotor experiences and caring human contact. During my time with Sasha, I helped him to develop and regulate his motor skills and learn to calm himself and focus his attention more effectively. Several years later, I had the opportunity to meet up with Sasha and his family. I found that Sasha's parents had formed a wonderful, caring, and nurturing relationship with him, and he was doing very well in school. Observing Sasha during a church service, he worked diligently to sit, stand, and kneel quietly. As the hour wore on, his small body began to gyrate ever so slightly. Tapping ensued, and, eventually, whole-body movements took over. Once it was absolutely impossible for him to remain still any longer, his parents had worked out a system where he was allowed to crawl over to a new location in the pew. This small physical transition was enough to refocus and calm him

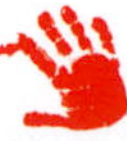

for the remainder of the service.

Sasha will always need to move around to stay focused. Long-distance running, learning karate, and playing hockey and other sports are likely activities that will help ensure his future success. With ongoing forms of sensory input that endeavors such as these can provide, he will be able to keep his neurological system well organized.

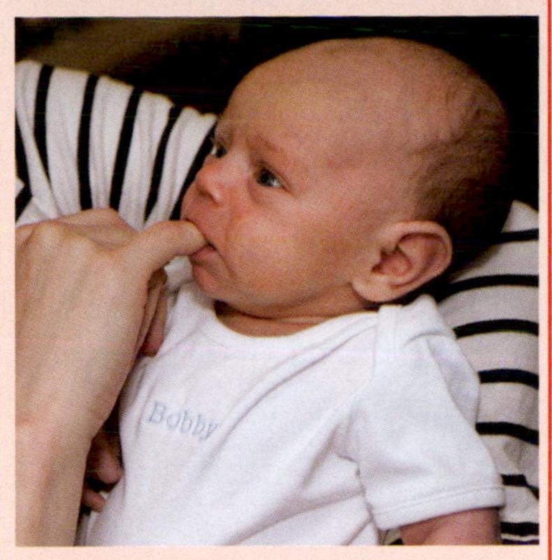

Figure 2. The sucking reflex. When a finger is placed on a newborn's lips, an automatic sucking motion occurs. This helps facilitate nursing soon after birth.

Hardwired for Movement

Newborns, although seemingly helpless, are hardwired to respond—albeit in a limited way—to the panoply of sensations that immediately follow birth. Newborn babies are equipped with primitive reflexes, which are preprogrammed movements made in response to specific stimuli. When touch and light pressure are applied to a newborn's lips, such as a bottle or

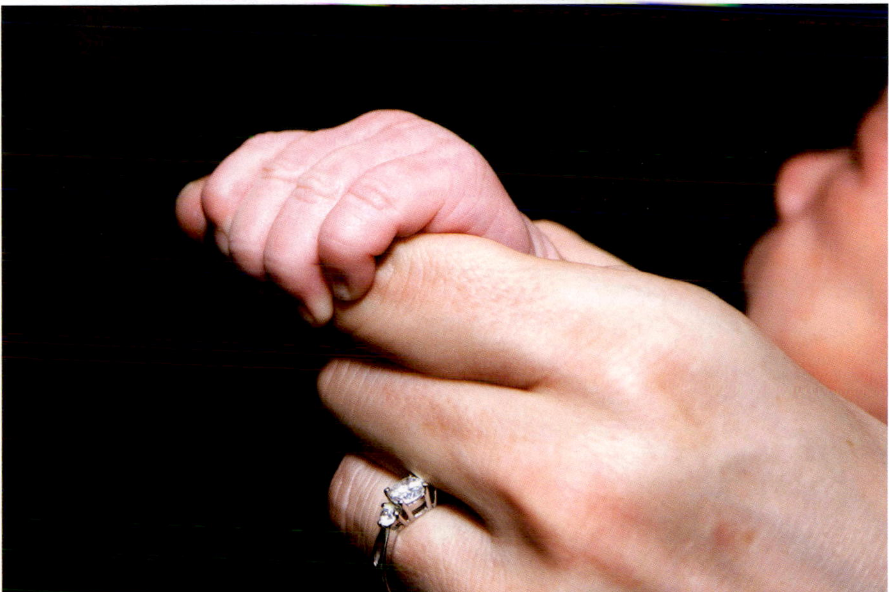

Figure 3. The grasping reflex. When an object is placed in the palm of an infant's hand, a squeezing or grasping motion occurs. The hold can be quite strong.

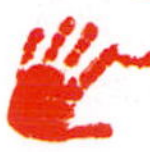

breast nipple, an immediate sucking motion occurs. This is called the sucking reflex **(Figure 2)**. Additionally, a variety of tactile, visual, and auditory stimuli facilitate movement in a young infant. Stroking the corner of the mouth outward to the cheek causes the tongue and head to move toward the stimulus. Introducing the nipple to the right or left side of a baby's lips will lead to him moving his head to the side. His neck muscles activate and start to build important connections between his head and his body.

When confronted with sudden movement or loud sounds, a young infant reacts with a total-body movement. His hands open wide, and he cries. This startle reflex occurs naturally in all babies. The response reflects the terror and discomfort the baby experiences when startled by unexpected, new, and sudden sensations. It is not recommended that you intentionally facilitate this uncomfortable response. This startle reflex is a primitive survival mechanism that, in addition to total-muscle activation, stimulates a stress reaction that unsettles the baby.

A more organizing reflex seen immediately after birth is the grasping reflex **(Figure 3).** When an object—typically a finger—is placed on a baby's palm, his fingers close tightly around it. This begins to activate muscles in his hand and allows him to interact with his caregiver in a very limited way.

Table 1. Primitive Reflexes in Newborns

Reflex	Stimulus	Action	Duration
Sucking reflex	Touch to the lips	Automatic sucking response	0-3 months
Grasping reflex	Touch to the palm	Hand closing around the source of the touch	0-3 months
Startle reflex	Sudden unpleasant stimulus	Abrupt total-body movement	0-3 months

Studies have shown that babies respond to a mother's voice and recognize her face within a few hours of life. When spoken to in pleasing tones, a baby will gaze intensely at her caregiver. If the caregiver changes to a new position, the baby's gaze will follow. This begins the development of visual tracking with the eyes.

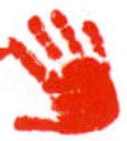

Imagine the joy of having your newborn meet your gaze, trying to figure out who you are and what you're about. What's in a gaze? Child psychiatrist Stanley Greenspan and the fabled pediatric expert T. Berry Brazelton discuss the importance of emotional connectivity from birth. Gazing at your infant helps establish that connection. Greenspan and Brazelton's research has shown that newborns actually attempt to keep themselves under control to be able to look at and listen to the caregivers around them. Visual images, such as a parent's face, soft voices, and gentle touch all help to regulate the infant and maintain an alert state.[1] These early moments form the basis of a lifelong relationship. A nurturing and loving relationship between parent and child provides the substrate for learning and the child's ability to establish a sense of self.

In those early moments, an unwritten contract can be established: Clause 1 states, "I am here for you, I will feed you, and I will try to protect you from those scary feelings and sounds." Clause 2 might say, "I will try to make these sights, sounds, and feelings more interesting and fun for you. I will challenge you to stay with me so we can explore and fully engage in the world together."

Peter Wolf and Heinz Prechtle identity six stages of consciousness in newborns:[2]

1. In the *quiet alert state,* the baby is responsive and focuses on an individual when spoken to. The baby's body is relaxed, and the eyes are attentive. The baby is very receptive in this state. This as an excellent time to deepen your relationship with your baby.
2. In the *active alert state,* the baby demonstrates rhythmic body movements, such as moving his legs or arms. This is an infant's way of interacting.
3. In the *drowsy state*, the eyes may be opened or closed. They are not focused. This is the state between wakefulness and sleep. It is not a time to disturb your baby for active engagement.
4. The *quiet sleep state* is when your baby sleeps quietly.
5. The *active sleep state* is when your baby moves around, much as you do while dreaming or during rapid eye-movement, or REM, sleep.

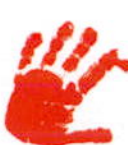

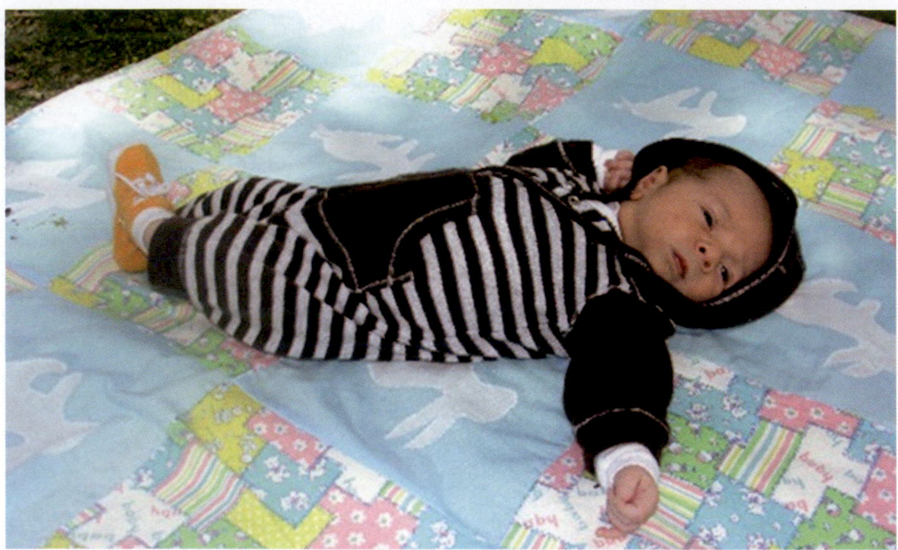

Figure 4. The fencing reflex. As the baby's head moves, one arm straightens or extends in the same direction as the head movement.

6. The *crying state* is your infant's way of communicating discomforts and needs, such as hunger or wanting a hug.

Soon after birth, when your infant appears to be in a quiet alert or active alert state, playing with your baby by dangling toys and making sounds will elicit her visual and listening attention. Touching and moving her in certain ways will jump-start early movement development.

Infants come into the world with "hardwired" motor responses, such as the grasping reflex discussed earlier. By touching the palm of her hand with your finger, your baby's hand closes tightly around your finger. Similarly, moving one of her arms in a certain direction, placing her in one position or another, or touching her skin in specific ways triggers specific movement patterns called *primitive reflexes*, just as the sucking occurred when her mouth was stimulated and her fist clenched when touch was applied to her hand. In healthy individuals, these reflexes fade away as intentional movement develops. Early on, however, when an infant is quite helpless, these reflexes provide a platform for early movement of her trunk and limbs. They facilitate movement in the baby. Although that little bundle needs total support, her muscles are already wired up to start moving in a limited way.

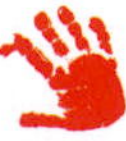

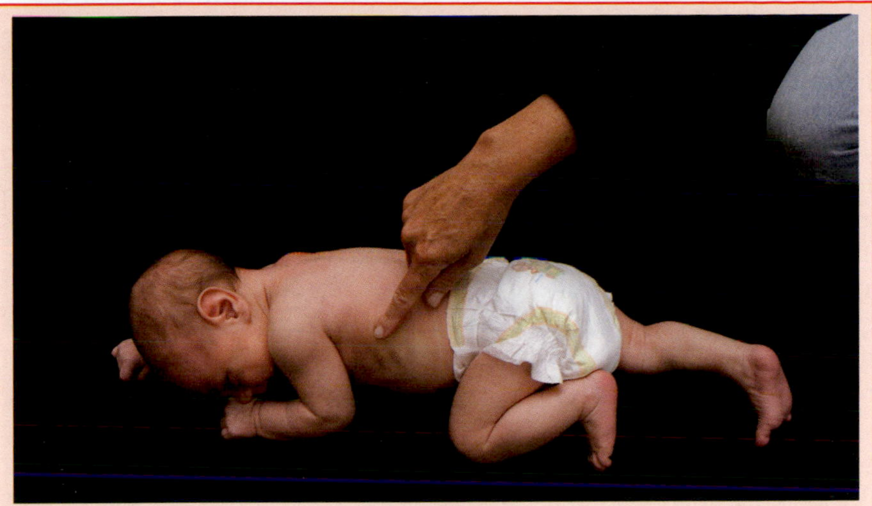

Figure 5. Stroking the baby's ribcage on the side of the trunk stimulates the Galant reflex, where the trunk bends in a curve like a "C."

There are many ways to encourage these primitive reflexes in that floppy little body.

Imagine Zorro at the ready, with his sword pointed outward, his right arm fully extended and his left arm artfully flexed over his shoulder, shouting, "En garde!" Now imagine a helpless little baby lying in her cradle, unknowingly mimicking this pose when an interesting sight, sound, or touch appears in her peripheral field. Her head will turn toward the stimulus. As her head moves, her arm straightens or extends in the same direction as her head movement. Her other arm bends upward toward the back of her head. This is called the fencing reflex **(Figure 4)**. The movement is primarily involuntary, but it begins to exercise the flexion and extension muscles in her arms and establishes an eye-hand connection as her head and eyes are directed toward her outstretched hand. If you gently extend her arm, the same response occurs. Her head turns in the direction of her extended arm, while her other arm bends toward her head.

Stroking or tickling your baby between his rib cage and his hip while he's lying in a prone position (on his stomach) causes his little trunk to bend in a curve like a "C." This is called lateral trunk flexion, or the Galant reflex. The movement activates muscles that wrap around his trunk, connecting the front and back of his body **(Figure 5)**.

Coordinated use of the muscles in the front and the back

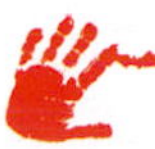

of the trunk leads to the ability to rotate, twist, and turn the body. We use rotation when turning around to look behind us—for instance, when backing up a car. Most sports require rotation—baseball, golf, and tennis are obvious examples. Everyday activities, such as picking something up off the floor, keeping yourself balanced in a car as it careens around a corner, and reaching up high to retrieve an object in a cabinet, all require use of these muscles.

Two-week-old infants are not ready to do abdominal exercises. However, the simple input administered to your baby when you're lifting him up can facilitate the activation of his trunk flexor muscles, similar to those used when you do sit-ups. When you exert some pressure on your baby's thighs while gently lifting and bending his head forward, his little body automatically assumes a partial sitting position. This is called *automatic sitting* **(Figure 6)**.

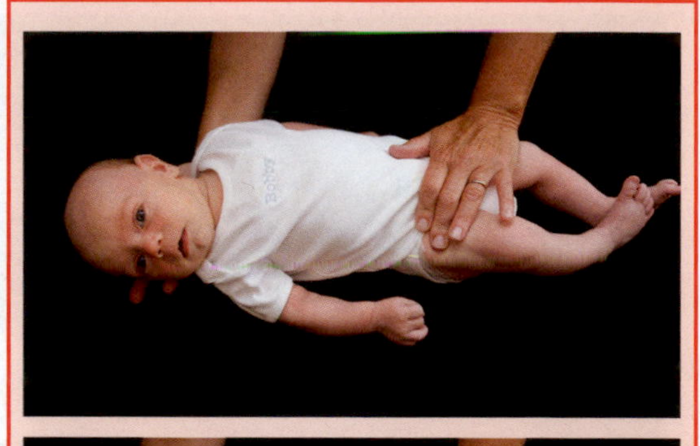

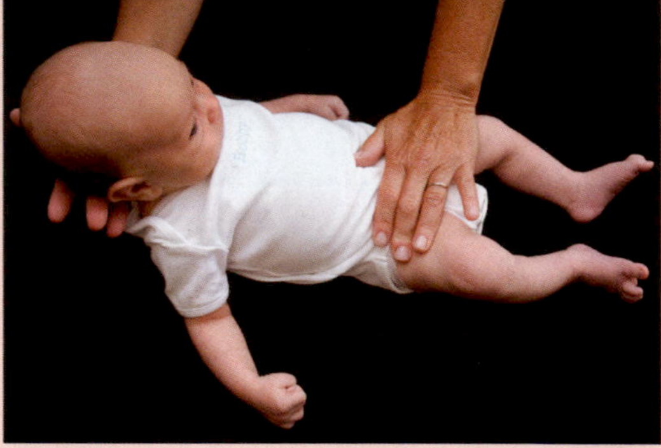

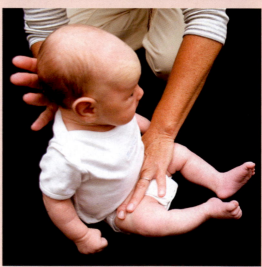

Figure 6. (a) To facilitate automatic sitting, gently apply pressure to the baby's hips and thighs and partially lift the head. **(b)** The baby will begin to activate muscles in the front of the neck and abdomen. **(c)** With assistance, the baby comes up to a supported sitting position.

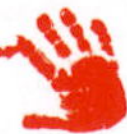

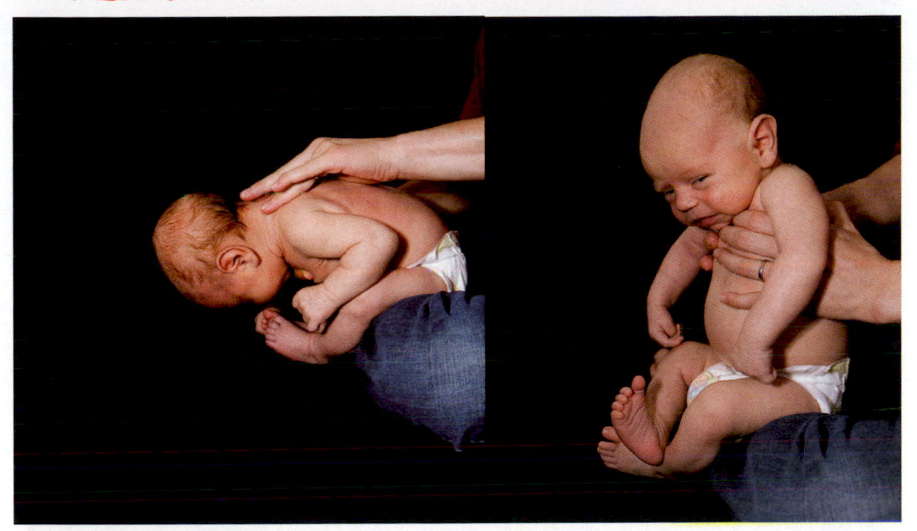

Figure 7. (a) Stroking the nape of a baby's neck stimulates the righting reaction. This leads to momentary extension of the neck, and the head lifts up. Strengthening the neck muscles helps develop head control. As the neck and back muscles strengthen, the infant can begin to assume an upright position, which facilitates easier exploration of the world. **(b)** As a result of stroking, the head and back momentarily lift, demonstrating the righting reaction.

While we do not and should not expect a baby to start a sit-up regime, the strengthening of the abdominal muscles is key to developing strong trunk muscles. We need these muscles to help us sit upright, pull ourselves up to stand, and provide a stable base from which other activities can derive, such as reaching for and manipulating objects.

Think of the many times your baby is lifted, moved, and repositioned—cradled in your arms, slung up onto your shoulder, or placed in his infant seat or back into his crib. When you're getting ready to move your baby, you can help him prepare by gently bending his head slightly and exerting pressure on his thighs. This stimulates his automatic sitting reflex, thereby activating his trunk muscles. Think of repositioning your baby as a cooperative process between you and your baby. Rather than using a swift, one-step motion, in which the baby is completely passive and helpless, consider it a transitional process, where you and your baby work as a team. When moving him from one location to another, if done slowly, in a supported and loving way, your baby's body awareness increases, and he gains confidence in making movement transitions.

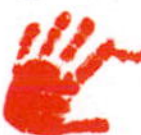

Strengthening your baby's back muscles is another critical aspect of healthy motor development. This process can also begin early by facilitating the righting reaction **(Figure 7)**. This is done by placing your baby in a squatting or sitting position on a firm surface, such as your thigh, with your baby's feet flat on the floor. By tickling or stroking the nape of his neck, momentary extension of his trunk and head occurs. Stimulating his neck and creating back extension is an alerting response, so your baby should be in an active alert stage when this is done. Because it is demanding to the neurological system, these "exercises" should only be done one or two times, and always preceded and followed by love and cuddles. Always remember to express affection to your baby—offer smiles and eye contact to reward your baby after these neurological exertions, no matter how small the movement may seem.

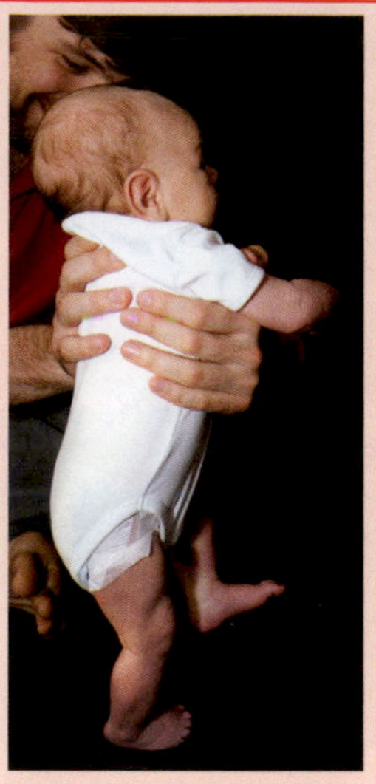

Figure 8. The stepping reflex. Holding the baby securely in an upright position while brushing the feet on a surface leads to a stepping movement in the baby's legs.

Another fun activity to try when your baby is in an active alert state is a type of precursor to walking. The stepping reflex can be facilitated by carefully holding your baby under her arms so she's in a standing position and inclining her trunk slightly forward, which causes a stepping motion to occur **(Figure 8).** While this does very little to strengthen her legs and does NOT lead to early walking, it sends information to her brain about her legs—"Hey, I'm here and ready to go!" This begins the building of motor pathways in your baby's brain. The more developed this "highway of information to the brain" is, the more efficient the transmission of sensorimotor information will be as your child grows.

Table 2. Primitive Reflexes Summary			
Reflex	Stimulus	Action	Duration
Fencing reflex	Turning the head or extending the arm	The head or arm follows	1-3 months
Galant reflex	Stroking the side of the trunk	The body curves	1-3 months
Sitting reflex	Applying pressure to the hips while gently flexing the neck	The trunk begins to try to sit up	1-3 months
Righting reaction	Stroking the nape of the neck while in the sitting position	The head lifts slightly	1-3 months
Stepping reflex	Tapping the foot on a firm surface while holding the baby in an upright position	A stepping motion occurs	1-3 months

Activating trunk-flexion and back-extension muscles begins the process of muscle strengthening that is so important for balancing and maintaining an upright position throughout the day. Being able to isolate limb movements, as occurs with the fencing reflex and the stepping reflex, sets the stage for being able to make voluntary movements of the arms and legs. The fencing reflex also sets up the eye-hand connection, as the head follows the movement of the arm.

With all of these reflexive patterns, engaging in these stimulating activities should be done judiciously. They should only be attempted when your baby is alert and "ready for action." Your infant should feel secure and have your full attention, so the movement is coupled with the give and take of play, such as pretend-dancing in the case of the stepping reflex. Establishing close physical contact, coupled with eye contact and positive verbal banter, helps make this a pleasurable experience for your baby.

How would you incorporate these activities into everyday life? The time you spend at the changing table is an opportune time to play with your baby. After you've changed her diaper and she is clean and calm, gently massage her limbs and stroke the side of her torso to activate her muscles and start building the pathways she needs to help organize her brain. As you lift her off the changing table, apply slight pressure to her thighs

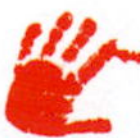

and gently flex her head forward. This will activate the sitting reflex.

As you sit on the floor to play with her, many of these reflexes can be stimulated. Dangle a toy to your baby's side while she is lying on her back (in the supine position), and see if her fencing reflex is activated. Prop her up on your leg in a supported sitting position, and stroke the back of her neck. Watch to see if her little head lifts up. Hold her in an upright position on a blanket and see if she looks like a miniature marathon runner as her little legs move.

These reflexes exemplify a few of the many primitive reflexes the human is equipped with at (or soon after) birth to be able to respond to the world. In normal development, these fade quickly. Timing varies, but they are usually no longer seen by 3 or 4 months old. You do not need to become a pediatric clinician to activate these specific body reflexes. Understand, however, that holding your baby in a variety of supported positions, moving your baby, and encouraging your baby to move throughout his or her waking hours will facilitate healthy development of the sensorimotor system.

Recommended Activities

When your child is startled, provide soothing and calming input. The number one priority is to make your infant feel safe and secure in this new world.

Calming strategies include the following:

- Using a soft voice
- Gentle bouncing and/or rocking
- Providing softer lights
- Using a gentle but firm hold
- Creating a less stimulating visual field
- Gentle but firm rubbing
- Changing positions (eg, holding your baby vertically against your body)
- Walking
- Gentle but firm stroking

When your baby is calm and alert, stimulating motor activity can be fun for all.

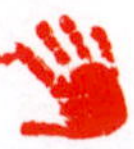

Never do these activities in a drill format. These should be part of an interplay of talking/babbling, making eye contact, and giving loving hugs. Less is more. Stimulating these reflexive responses should occur only once or twice, with a big break in between. The thrill of success the baby experiences from your rapturous response to each little effort will do more for her confidence and willingness to take risks later on than trying to do 10 reps and ending up with a fussy and exhausted infant.

Light touch causes hyperalerting of the nervous system and can make your baby fussy. Gentle but firm pressure will provide positive input to stimulate the muscles in her trunk. Using techniques such as infant massage provides soothing ways to wake up her skin and trunk muscles.

Consider repositioning your infant as a transitional process rather than an instantaneous occurrence. For example, transition your baby from lying in a supine position to a supported sitting position by slowly lifting her head and supporting her thighs, then lifting her up to a full sitting position.

Initiate and follow each effort with positive responses and firm physical support, so your baby feels safe and successful.

Movement for Organization

During the first 3 months of my son's life, he "preferred" being held in an upright position and recognized immediately when I sat down, even though I took great care to keep holding him the same way. Somehow the gentle rock or bounce I provided while standing felt different than when I was sitting. Much to my chagrin, he was quite intractable to any change, particularly when he was tired. As a pediatric therapist, I knew that during his active alert states I could place him on his stomach for tummy time and other positions. When he was tired, all bets were off, and the only way to soothe him was by using the "standing vertical hold." The music of Cindy Lauper and U2 helped him fall asleep, but the moment I ever-so-gently placed him down in his crib, he'd wake up—wailing.

Your baby may love to be cradled horizontally in your arms, and you may love the serenity of rocking him peacefully in this position all day. But your child needs to experience

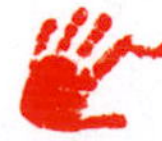

other positions, as well. Holding him in a vertical position and placing him briefly on his tummy enables him to tolerate new movements and positions comfortably. And a comfortable baby is a calmer, happier baby.

Positioning your baby in a variety of postures, such as placing him on his back (supine) or on his stomach (prone), lying on his side, sitting in a supported sitting position, and standing, is important for many reasons. As long as his head is always well supported, these positions are another way to teach him about the world and experience new sensations inside his body. Many movements and positions, such as the primitive reflexes we've discussed, can stimulate muscle activity in his body, which precedes intentional movement. In addition to this, depending on the position he is placed in, he will begin to experience new feelings and sensations. When movement is also provided, whether it be gentle rocking, bouncing, or "flying" through the air, his brain begins to learn about these sensations of movement and helps your baby become comfortable in the world.

Feeling where the body rests in space occurs because of a "quiet sense" called proprioception. Without opening our eyes, we know if we are sitting or standing. Our sensors for proprioception are located in our joints and muscles. When stimulated, these nerve cells send a message up to our brain. This information then travels to the parts of the brain that coordinate movement. While some hardwiring is present, a child fully develops this body sense through life experiences. The sooner a child experiences new positions, the sooner critical connections will be made to help develop the internal mapping of body awareness.

Movement stimulates another "silent" or "internal" sense, called kinesthesia. "Kinetics" relates to movement, and kinesthesia refers to the sensation of moving. One knows or feels that an arm or leg has moved without having to see the actual movement. Over time, an individual learns exactly how many inches to move an arm when reaching for a glass without looking. My son apparently had an acute sense of body position and movement, as he was able to discern the difference in rocking while I stood versus when I was seated!

To understand proprioception on the high end of the athletic spectrum, a good tennis player feels exactly how to angle his or

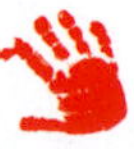

her wrist when hitting the ball to a specific location on the court. Feeling the correct wrist position results from finely tuned proprioception. Knowing how much force to exert when hitting the ball comes from a highly developed sense of movement, or kinesthesia.

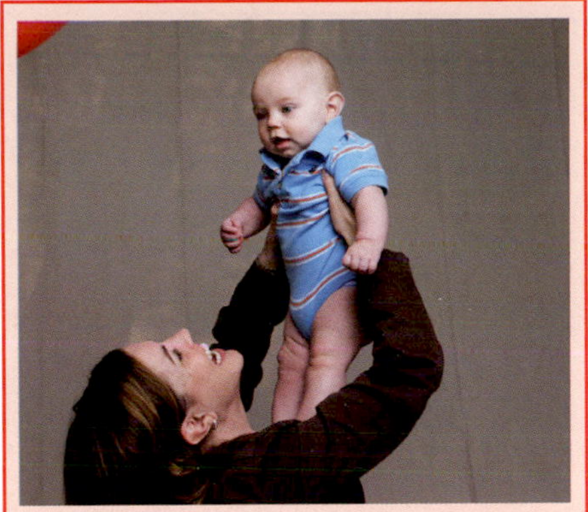

Figure 9. Mixing it up with movement. At 5 months old, Bobby is able to hold his head up securely, so faster movement play can occur with less support. These same activities were done when he was younger, but more support was given and the pacing was much slower.

The vestibular system, the third internal sense organ, is linked to detecting motion, such as spinning and moving fast. We become aware of our vestibular systems when we get dizzy after a roller coaster ride or seasick on a boat. In these instances, the vestibular system has been overloaded. Some people crave rotation in all forms: amusement park rides, sailing on the high seas, and spinning like a dancer or figure skater. While they might not realize why, they crave these activities because their vestibular systems prefer a high degree of stimulation. Others avoid such activities, as the circular motion

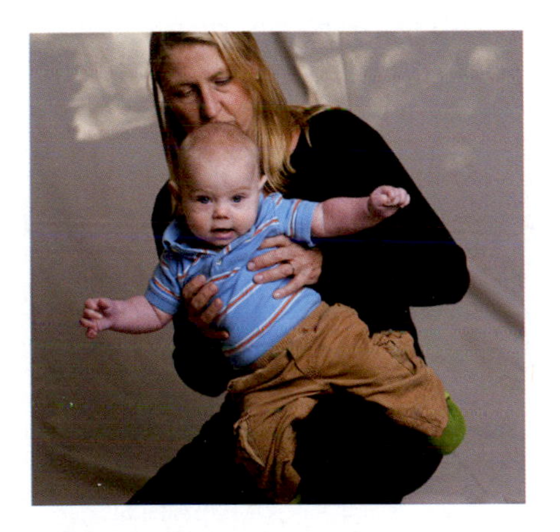

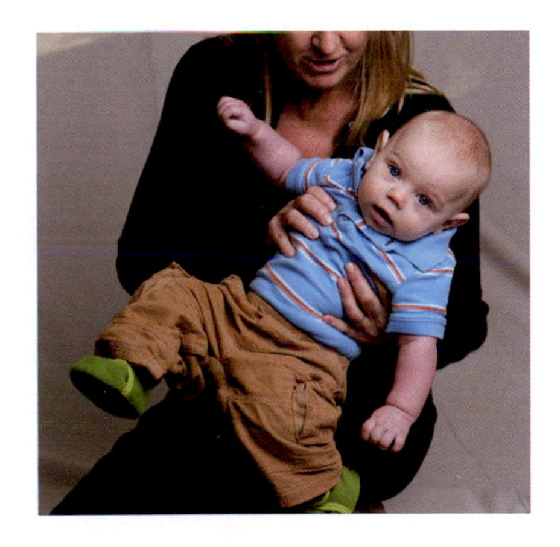

Figure 10. (a) I did these same bouncing and rocking movements with Bobby when he was an infant, by supporting him against my chest. **(b)** Now that he has better head and trunk control, he needs less support, and the muscles in his body can do the work.

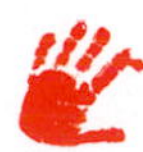

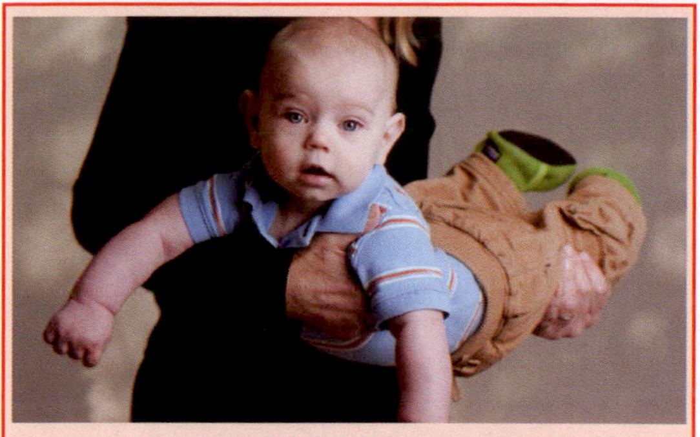

Figure 11. When "flying" as an infant, one of my arms supported the length of Bobby's trunk, while my other arm gave extra support to his upper body and head. He frequently sucked my thumb while that support was given.

makes them sick. These individuals have more sensitive or hypersensitive vestibular systems.

The vestibular system also helps us detect "linear" motion, or our speed and direction when moving in a straight line. We generally do not need to look out the car window to determine whether the car is moving and when it is going fast or slow. The vestibular system is responsible for this innate understanding of the direction and speed of movement. Coupling the information from the muscles and joints (kinesthetic/proprioceptive system) with the information from the vestibular system, your baby begins to learn where her body is in space—upside down, rocking, bouncing, or falling!

Activating all of these sensory systems is very important for your baby to be able to learn about the world and gain a better sense of how her little body moves in space. So, playfully engaging her in varied movement is very healthy and important, as long as her head is well supported **(Figures 9-11)**.

Table 3. The Quiet Senses

Sense	Activation	Function
Proprioception	Pressure to the joints	Senses where body parts are
Kinesthesia	Movement of the muscles	Detects movement of the body parts
Vestibular sense	Rotation and movement; change in head position	Interprets movement of the whole body: spinning, rocking, direction, and speed of movement

Beyond providing a recognition of falling, which has obvious survival value, the proprioceptive/kinesthetic/vestibular triad

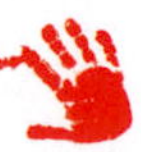

has significant influence in the development of your baby's brain. In many ways, parts of the brain reflect the complex workings of a train station. Imagine tracks merging, incoming trains, outgoing trains, and the need for a central system to organize all of it. The human brain receives billions of impulses every second, so it needs to figure out what to pay attention to and what to ignore. This selection of information occurs constantly. Depending on the level of alertness and sophistication of the brain, this sorting of "necessary" and "unnecessary" information occurs continuously. Typically, babies have immature neurological organization, so they do not filter this information overload very well. As a result, they can get overstimulated very easily.

Stimulation from the silent senses turns on "inhibitory neurons" in the brain. These nerve cells act to "extinguish" or switch off the nerve signals from input entering the brain that is not useful at any given time. The more of these inhibitory nerve cells that are activated, the more efficient and organized the brain becomes in processing all of the sensations bombarding it.

To understand how this occurs, draw your attention to how your feet feel when touching the floor. It is likely that until you read those words, you were unaware of the feeling of pressure created by your feet resting on the floor. If the floor suddenly began to vibrate because of an earthquake, your brain would automatically switch attention to this incoming sensation and then alert your entire system to organize a motor response, such as running to exit the building or finding a safe doorjamb to protect yourself from impending damage. If you are wearing shoes that fit too tightly, you may have already been aware of your feet because your brain received a message that blood flow was constricted or that your skin was abraded from the poor fit.

We usually think of "paying attention" as a fairly active, higher-level thinking task. But way before language and formal thought develop, your baby's neurological system is forming the substrate of networks necessary to maintain efficient focus and attention. This neurological organization helps foster the efficient transmission of information necessary for coordinated gross-motor ability and the ability to efficiently combine and sort out all kinds of visual, tactile, auditory, and moving experiences.

Toddlers with a history of prematurity and multiple medical conditions are frequently referred to me. During those critical

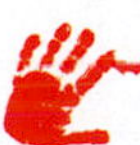

first months of life, the premature infant is poked and probed with needles, tubes, harsh lights, and distracting sounds. Opportunities to be cuddled, bounced, and rocked are limited by the necessary life-and-death struggle that affects the child daily. Along with the painful sensations interwoven into the child's struggle for survival, the supportive input that calms the nervous system and facilitates healthy growth is often absent.

Consider Ashley. She was born 2 months early and weighed 2 pounds 3 ounces at birth. Her lungs had not matured, so breathing assistance was required to keep her alive. A feeding tube constituted her sole source of nutrition for the first 2 years of her life. The tube was placed in her abdomen, causing her extreme discomfort if pressure or pulling were accidentally inflicted on the site. So much for tummy time when playing! Most of Ashley's first 6 months was spent lying on her back, attached to a series of tubes in an incubated cradle. Any movement at all would inflict discomfort or pain.

Ashley was referred to me at 2 years old by her pediatrician because she was hypersensitive to touch and movement. She had just learned to walk but was fearful whenever a surface was uneven. She was terrified of falling. She resisted any new form of movement. Toddler swings, merry-go-rounds, and unfamiliar cars became objects of dread. While Ashley occasionally tolerated a stroller, she mostly insisted on being held. In the clothing department, she wore only one outfit and refused to wear anything else. This necessitated Mom having to wash Ashley's clothes each night, no matter how exhausted she might be. Presenting little Ashley with a different set of clothes would lead to a tantrum of unknown duration. Tantrums led to breathing difficulties. The pulmonologist had cautioned against allowing tantrums to transpire.

This adorable little girl had missed the opportunity to enjoy movement and the exploration of touch, which most infants experience naturally. Her nervous system had mostly learned that any stimulus inflicts pain and discomfort. As a result, almost all sensory stimuli led to having a stress response. Being held in her mommy's arms was the only line of defense she felt she had.

Very gradually, Ashley was introduced to many forms of movement and tactile experiences. When her feeding tube

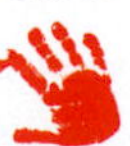

was removed, she began working the muscles in her tummy, and the strength in her back developed. Falling onto soft surfaces, such as pillows and mats, became a fun experience rather than a life-threatening one. Ashley gained a better sense of how her body moved and began to trust that she had the ability to protect herself from injury as she moved around. As her nervous system gained experience in accepting touch input, she became more flexible in what she could wear. The terror responses that had previously occurred multiple times a day diminished. Her family began to go on outings together, as uncontrollable outbursts were no longer a problem. Many activities done during treatment sessions were integrated into Ashley's daily schedule. Over time, these games became a natural part of her play routines. We all knew that Ashley was on a healthy track when she began playing dress-up with her big sister, wrapping a feathery boa around her body and climbing up on the coffee table (serving as a pretend "runway") to exhibit the latest in haute couture.

Your instinctive impulse to rock or bounce your baby, along with cooing and stroking, sends messages to that organizing part of your baby's brain. It stimulates the development of nerve pathways that make up an "organization matrix." Every parent discovers that this wondrous little being enjoys or craves certain movements, such as being bounced or rocked. You may discover even faster the ones your baby dislikes. This does not mean that you should avoid such movements forever. It simply requires a more gradual introduction of the movement over time. For example, your baby may love to be walked and bounced, but when rocked in a chair (which gives you some relief!), your child stiffens and screams. Alternating a bounce, bounce, rock, rock, and mixing up sitting and standing for short durations will help your child learn to tolerate and eventually enjoy both sensations. This may occur in one evening, or it may take several months.

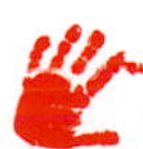

Recommended Activities

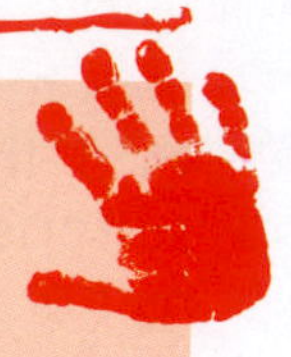

Ways to activate proprioceptors:

- Gentle bouncing
- Massaging muscles
- Applying gentle pressure at the shoulders and hips

Ways to activate kinesthetic and vestibular receptors:

- Walking your baby
- Rocking your baby
- Swinging your baby
- Taking car rides
- Introducing gentle rotation
- Gently moving your baby's limbs, fingers, and toes
- Gently tipping your baby forward, backward, and side to side while well supported

Positioning for Strength and Control

Concerns about Sudden Infant Death Syndrome resulted in counseling families to have infants sleep on their backs. This keeps the air passages fully open. As this has become the recommended position for sleeping, your child needs to spend more time in other positions during waking hours. Placing your baby on a blanket, tummy-side down, activates his neck and back muscles. These are critical for strengthening the core muscles in his trunk, which are so important for developing motor control. Propping his back against a cushion allows him to lie on his side. This stretches the muscles around the sides of his body.

When you get down with your child to play, shaking rattles or making silly faces and noises to gain his visual attention, eventually he will lift his head to look at the hullabaloo. Over time, as his interest grows for grown-up antics, his arms will come forward to push his head slightly higher for a better view.

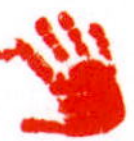

This strengthens his neck, back, arm, and hand muscles even further.

Positioning to Increase Core Strength

Prone: Your baby is placed on his tummy. A pillow can be used to prop up your baby's chest.

Side Lying: Your baby is placed on his side, with a pillow propped against his back for support.

Supported Sitting: Your baby is placed on your lap, while you provide support through his trunk and head as needed.

Supine: Your baby is placed on his back; this is passive, so it is important to engage him in "looking" activities and eventually "reaching" activities when he's in this position.

Sitting your child upright, supported in your lap, while gently moving him side to side and back and forth, provides further positional and moving cues. Leaning him backward ever so slightly while supporting his head and maintaining visual attention, your child works hard to hold your gaze. This exercises his neck and eye muscles and develops head control. As your baby becomes more adventurous and you become more confident in supporting his head and trunk safely, using increased vigor in rocking, swinging, and gentle twirling motions can bring great pleasure to the baby and to you. Mutual admiration will develop as these sensory-rich personal encounters occur throughout your baby's waking day.

Several years ago, I visited an old college buddy who had recently had a baby. My children, in their late teens, sat terrified at dinner as they watched the dad swing and flip his 6-month-old daughter, Amanda, in the air. I assured them that I was thrilled to see my friend provide all that kinesthetic and vestibular input

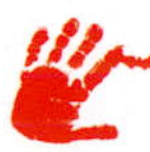

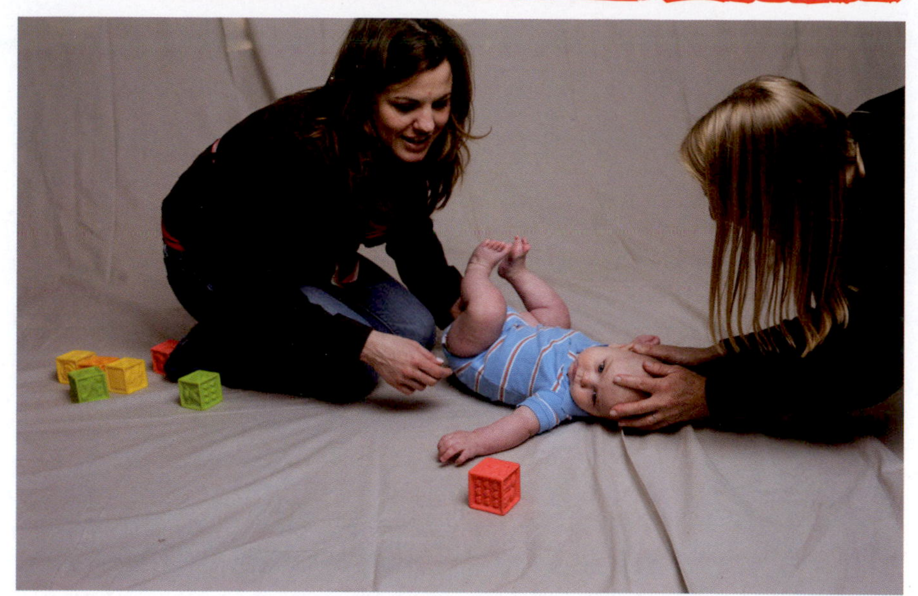

Figure 12. The neck-righting reaction. The head is gently turned to the side, and the body follows. **Caution:** Babies do not enjoy this movement! I **do not** recommend that you try this reaction with your baby.

and predicted the child would be quite a "star." Fast-forward 3 years. My friend came to visit, and this little "star" outperformed my expectations. At the age of 3, Amanda was highly verbal, attentive, and quite agile in her fine- and gross-motor abilities. We spent one morning picking wild blueberries. Not only was she able to discriminate between ripe and unripened fruit, she also used a refined pincer grasp and managed to work her way among the scrubby bushes with ease. My attention span and stamina for the task waned long before hers did.

While it's a huge leap to link all of Amanda's accomplishments to the aerial feats executed in her first year, this sensory input no

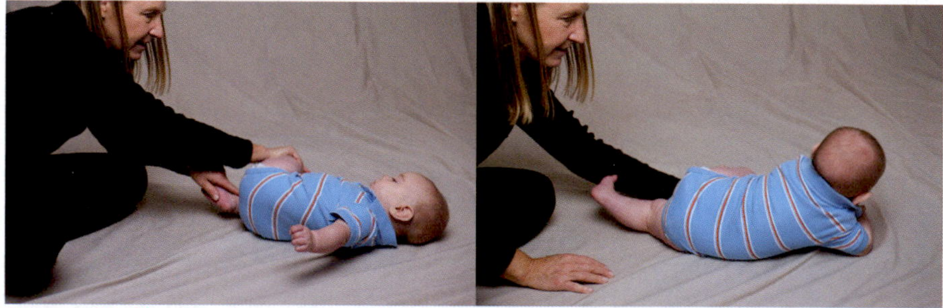

Figure 13. The body-on-body righting action. **(a)** The leg is gently moved up toward the trunk and across the other leg. **(b)** As the first leg crosses over the other, the body follows.

doubt helped organize her neurological system. Since she was comfortable and flexible with all kinds of sensory stimulation, she was "available" for attending to language games and had the concentration to work through challenging visual-motor tasks, such as puzzles and block structures. Amanda had developed a strong body sense and confidence in tackling all kinds of gross- and fine-motor challenges.

Along with the hardwired primitive reflexes seen at birth, babies have other automatic movements that develop soon after. These help their little bodies move into a comfortable position if they find themselves in a precarious or uncomfortable situation. These movements are called automatic postural reactions, and they help infants to regain a comfortable position from an unbalanced or awkward one. The automatic postural reactions serve as a bridge from rigid motor responses to voluntary or intentional movements, which form the basis of all motor control.

When you turn a baby's head to one side, she experiences discomfort, and her body will follow to regain a position of comfort. This is called the neck-righting reaction, where the head and body move as a unit **(Figure 12)**.

Similarly, the *body-on-body righting reaction* occurs when the leg is shifted upward toward the trunk and across the other leg. The body follows and flips over. This begins to isolate leg movements and is a precursor to rolling **(Figure 13)**.

When your baby is placed on her stomach, the *labyrinth righting reaction* causes her head to lift up and possibly turn from side to side.

Table 4. Automatic Postural Reactions Summary

Reaction	Stimulus	Action
Neck-righting reaction	The head turns	The body follows
Body-on-body reaction	The leg moves across the opposite hip	The body follows and flips over
Labyrinth righting reaction	The baby is placed on her stomach	The head lifts up

As with primitive reflexes, you should not place your child on an exercise mat and attempt to begin a Pilates routine.

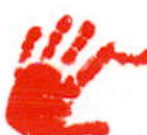

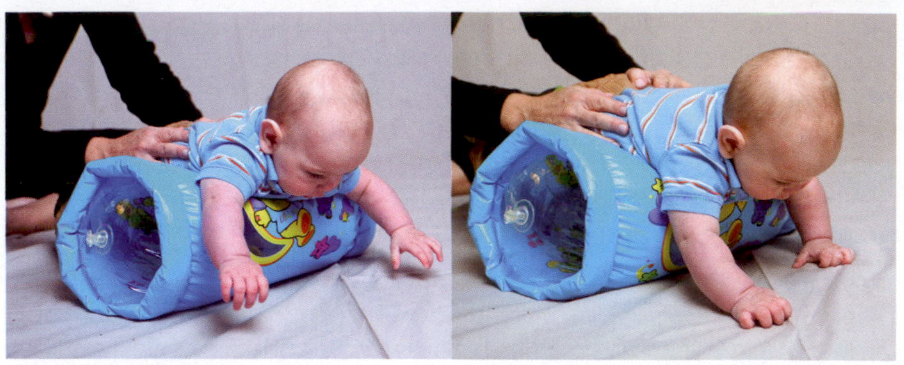

Figure 14. (a) Bobby enjoys rolling over this inexpensive inflatable toy and gently "crashing" to the floor. A soft, inflated play ball purchased at the grocery store can be used, as well. **(b)** Make sure this activity is done on a soft surface, such as on thick carpeting or couch cushions. The baby should have good head control before attempting activities like these.

Just as we discussed before, play with your baby during diaper changes and baths, and use playtime and daily routines to explore new ways to move your baby. Gentle movement and guidance of her limbs to the right and left, up and down, will help her gain body awareness and activate her trunk and limb musculature. Positioning your baby on her tummy, her side, and her back activates different muscle groups. These activities help her become familiar and comfortable with a variety of positions and movements. They lead to the many underpinnings necessary for skilled motor engagement that comes later in development.

While some children crave and delight in the novelty of movement and different body positions, others are tentative and resist initial efforts to try out new experiences. Some individuals thrive on the thrill of riding on the scariest roller coasters and in speeding cars. Others cringe at the idea of getting on a merry-go-round. Everyone's sensorimotor system has its own preferences. To be able to function properly, however, whether a "couch potato" or a world-class athlete, each person needs to be able to tolerate movement in a variety of ways. Without the tolerance for varied movements and the physical endurance to maintain healthy postures for extended periods, an individual may become anxious, overwhelmed, preoccupied, or exhausted when confronted with new motor sensations. This leads to fatigue and a lack of concentration for the demands of the surrounding environment, whatever they

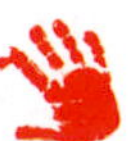

might be.

Therefore, it is important to gradually introduce a growing infant to a variety of motor experiences. Many have been reviewed in this chapter. Positioning a baby on her back, side, and tummy all help develop different muscle groups in her neck and trunk. Holding her in vertical, horizontal, and supported sitting positions also helps develop trunk strengthening. Finally, introducing movement of various forms, such as bouncing, rocking, and moving in different directions, gives a baby experiences that help develop flexibility of her neurological system and builds pathways for future motor learning **(Figure 14)**.

Recommended Activities

Positioning and movement can have a calming influence on your baby. Exploration of your baby's preferred positions and movement experiences helps strengthen your bond with your child. It can become a powerful tool in helping to regulate your child's comfort level, as well as encouraging engagement.

Before your child can cope with and begin to figure out what's going on in her surrounding environment, she needs to be calm and well regulated.

Facilitating movement starts to build:

- head and neck control
- coordinated motor responses
- eye contact
- eye-hand coordination

Engaging your child through eye contact, verbal exchange, and movement forms the bedrock for a positive parent-child relationship.

When your infant is calm, use the time together to have playful and rich sensorimotor interactions throughout the day.

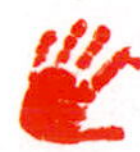

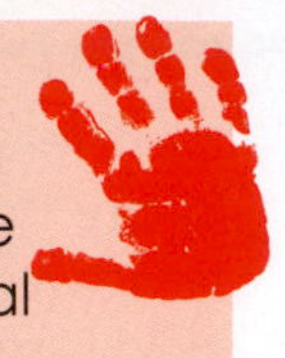

Incorporate soothing sounds, movements, positions, and touch input to encourage a sense of calm and engagement in your baby. Use more dynamic movements, sounds, and additional visual stimuli to provide challenging experiences.

With all interactions, either to soothe or to challenge, begin with and sustain eye contact, make the interactions fun, and always make sure your baby feels secure and loved.

Primitive reflexes and automatic reactions serve as a bridge to flexible and intentional movement. These early patterns should fade over time. If primitive reflexes and automatic reactions persist well past the time frame outlined in this chapter, discuss this with your pediatrician.

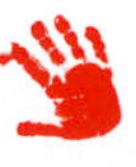

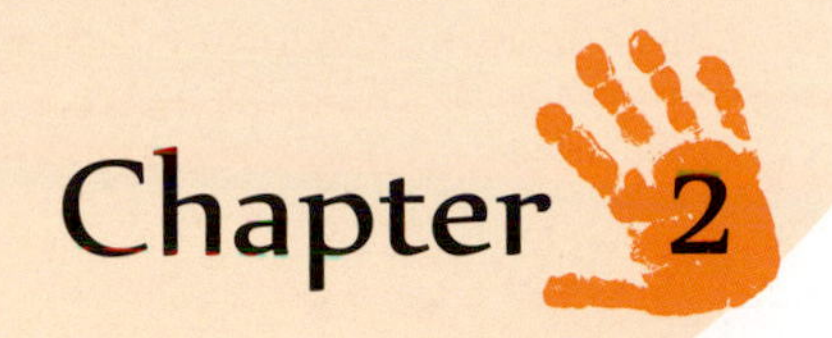

Chapter 2

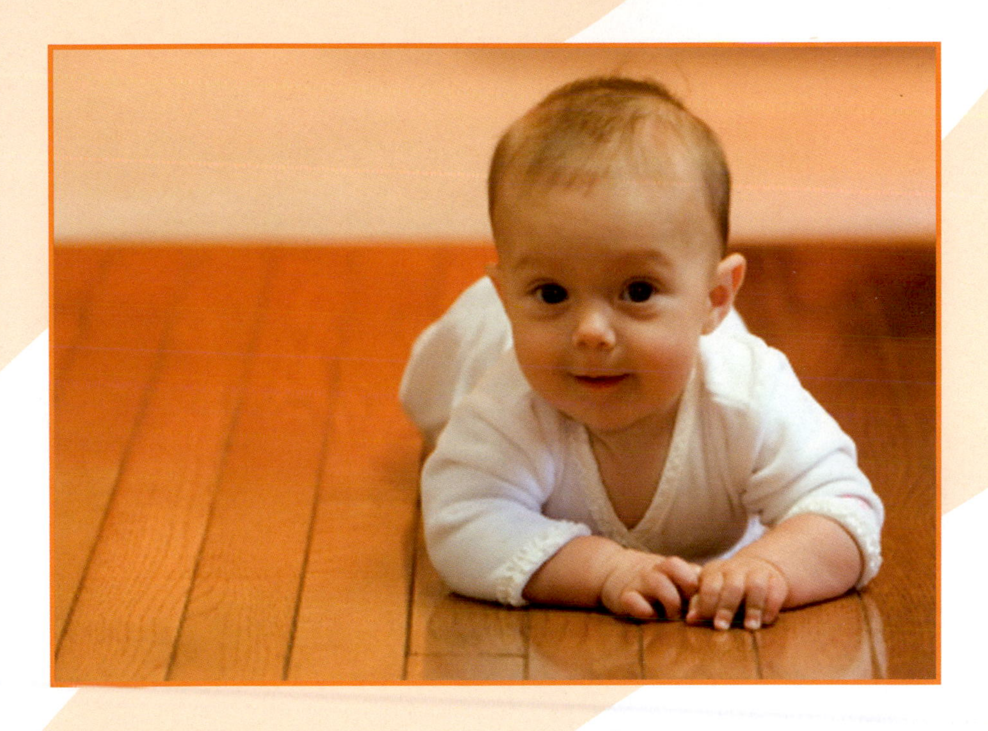

Movement through the First Year

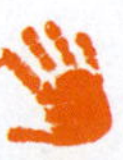

Sometimes, less is more. In the case of Ashley, less pain as a tiny infant would have led to more exploration. With Sasha, less neglect would have allowed him to receive the critical stimulation necessary for him to ensure a balanced sensory system. For Tommy, a little less coddling may have prevented delays in development that became apparent as his first year unfolded. Tommy was referred to me at 9 months old. The primary concern was that he experienced hypersensitivities to touch and appeared to be frequently frustrated.

Unlike Ashley, who experienced noxious stimuli throughout the first year of her life, or Sasha, who endured an absence of any stimulation, Tommy was doted upon—to the extreme. He had two loving parents and a nurse. Whenever Tommy whimpered, he was picked up and cuddled. As time went on, being an astute and intelligent infant, Tommy learned that each cry led to immediate comfort. The need to hold his head up or reach for a toy never occurred. As a result, Tommy never developed strong trunk and head control.

Because of his fussiness, Tommy was held and fully supported 24 hours a day. As a result, he never developed a tolerance for different positions, such as lying on his side or on his stomach. By the time he came to see me, Tommy was unable to sleep unless someone held him, and he cried whenever he was put down. He had just learned to assume a supported sitting position but was unable to reach for or play with toys because he needed both hands to keep his body upright. When support was provided for sitting, he still only used one hand to manipulate a toy. The other hand was always occupied with keeping himself balanced, whether necessary or not. As a result, Tommy had not acquired the ability to use both hands together to play.

Tommy needed to play catch-up in all aspects of his motor development. Using the mantra "No pain, *no pain*" was not serving his long-term interest. His body needed to get stronger so he could sit without support. Then both arms would be freed up to manipulate his toys. Tommy also needed to learn that moving in new ways could actually be a pleasurable experience.

Tommy's family was given a home program, with the following objectives:

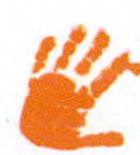

1. Learning how to position Tommy in a variety of ways: lying on his side, lying in a prone position, and supported sitting.
2. Providing enjoyable movement experiences: bouncing, rocking, and tipping him in different directions when sitting on someone's lap.
3. Providing touch experiences to increase his tolerance for varied sensory experiences. This included creating a tactile basket full of interesting textured objects (such as paintbrushes, hairbrushes, velvet, lambs' wool, and sandpaper).
4. Encouraging reaching to the sides to improve his trunk-rotation ability, as Tommy's trunk strength improved.

I observed Tommy 2 years later, when he entered preschool. Happily, he moved around the classroom comfortably and enjoyed the many fine-motor activities available to him, with both hands working together effectively. He was a well-adjusted, fully functioning preschooler.

Many parents look forward to their baby's tentative first steps, which occur somewhere around 12 months, as a major developmental accomplishment. Somewhere between birth and this magical moment, a motor transformation of enormous proportion occurs. This transformation begins with the reflexes discussed in the previous chapter. In this chapter, we'll look at when and how *intentional movement* begins. As your baby attempts to literally grasp at the world around him, many important things are happening to make him stronger and more coordinated.

At approximately 4 months of age, intentional movement truly establishes itself. As your baby's body gets stronger, reaching out to swat at a mobile becomes possible. This is a monumental event. It usually occurs without fanfare, but when your child intentionally stretches out a hand to touch a toy, it marks the beginning of cognitive and motor integration. Bilaterality, or the use of two hands together, also takes your child to a whole new level of interacting with his environment. When your baby learns to sit independently, so many important elements of motor control have been established that burgeoning independence soon follows. Crawling and pulling himself up to stand, if they are not already occurring, are practically moments away.

We will review how reaching, sitting, crawling, and using two hands develop and allow your child to interact with his surroundings in a purposeful way. We will also discuss how to encourage your growing baby to reach, sit, and crawl.

Intentional Movement Begins

When a baby sees an object and purposely moves toward it, several things are happening. To begin with, the child identifies the object as something "real." This means that a concept about the toy is developing. Curiosity leads to a desire to explore this item. The brain instructs the motor centers to organize a motor response—and voila! "Reaching out to touch something" occurs.

Up until this point, your baby's little limbs moved back and forth, up and down, pretty much in a random fashion. At various times, her hands brushed against objects. It may have been Daddy's scratchy face, the babysitter's finger, or all of the toys thrust in front of her by her big brother. Each of those moments of contact fed information to her brain, gradually forming into the concept that these images have a physical form and can be touched.

Her arm motions become more organized, and your baby develops a sense of how to direct the movements. When observing your infant in the very early stages of batting at toys, trial and error is the overriding element. She may look intently at the object and then make a few seemingly random swipes toward it. Depending on the temperament of your baby and her energy level at any given time, her flailing arm may continue to work doggedly until contact is made. Once she succeeds, the enjoyment of watching the cause and effect of touching the object usually motivates her to continue playing this game.

Each time she succeeds in hitting the toy, her eye-hand connection develops. A growing awareness of how to move her arm occurs, and her accuracy increases.

Swatting at a mobile or reaching for a toy has many benefits. Extending her arm develops shoulder stability and continues strengthening her trunk. As her eyes direct her arm, eye-hand coordination begins to take root.

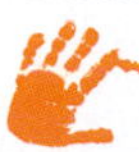

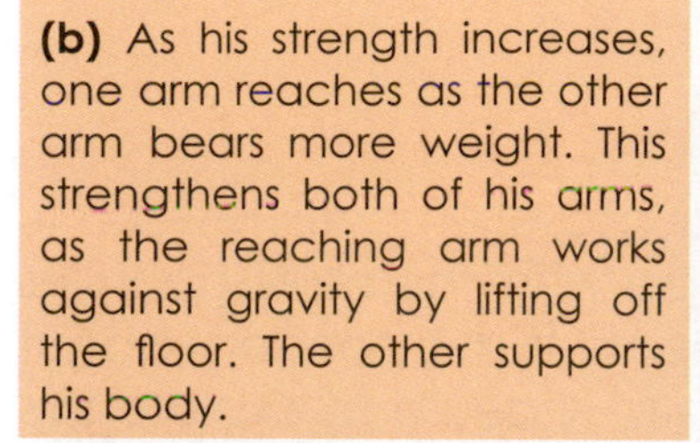

Figure 15. (a) As his back and arms get stronger, Bobby is able to prop himself up on his elbows to lift his head.

(b) As his strength increases, one arm reaches as the other arm bears more weight. This strengthens both of his arms, as the reaching arm works against gravity by lifting off the floor. The other supports his body.

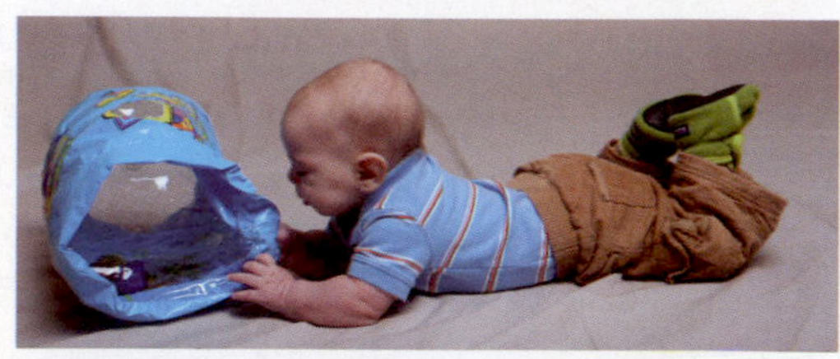

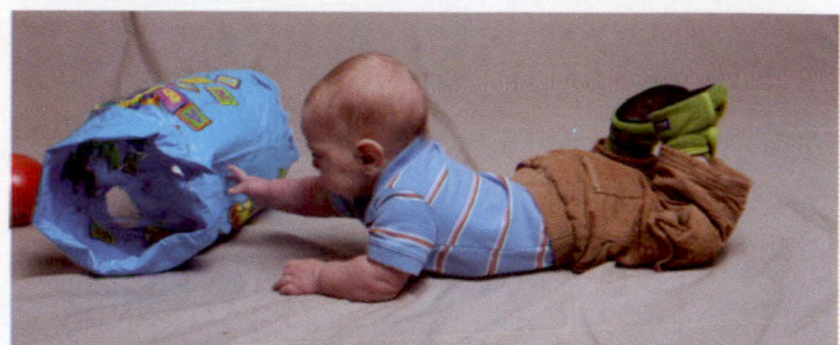

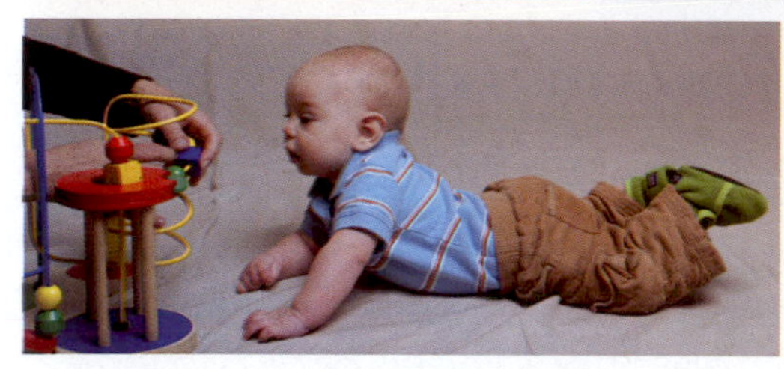

Figure 16. One day, a baby will be strong enough to lift his chest up off the floor. His arms straighten, and his weight is now borne by his hands. Fascinated by a new toy, Bobby lifts himself up higher to get a closer look.

When your baby is able to explore toys strategically placed on a blanket during floor play, more time spent looking at and touching the objects can occur. As she attempts to grasp a toy beyond her reach, her legs may flex up, facilitating movement forward or an inadvertent rollover. This, in turn, may result in successful acquisition of the toy, which is a powerful experience in autonomy.

The inadvertent act of rolling over or scooting forward may become a delight in itself and leads to experimentation with this new movement. She attempts to repeat the motion until she learns to roll or scoot successfully.

You can encourage reaching and moving. Place a toy truck in front of her during tummy time. Her head will lift to observe the vehicle. Curiosity usually leads to reaching. If her immediate interest is not sparked, move the vehicle back and forth, making "beeping" sounds to entice her. Once she is engaged, push the truck back a little farther than her arm can reach. This requires her to make a bigger movement to obtain the toy. As her arm stretches farther, her shoulder and back muscles become engaged. Push the toy closer, if necessary, to make sure she successfully makes contact with it. The effort to reach should be rewarded! Make a big deal about the accomplishment…big efforts demand big praise **(Figures 15 and 16)**.

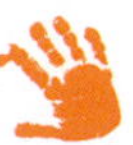

The progression of tummy work can be intriguing to watch!

1. Your baby lifts her head to observe her surroundings. Over time, curiosity demands a broadening of her visual field, which necessitates a higher stance.
2. Gradually, your child pushes her body and head higher, creating an arch in her back. Initially, the weight of her upper trunk is borne in her forearms and elbows.
3. Her arms are used vigorously to push her body off the floor. This action results in heavy weight-bearing in her arms and hands. Weight-bearing strengthens her muscles and facilitates an awareness or feeling in her joints. Nerve cells located in her joints are stimulated. These send a signal up to her brain, which in turn connects to the areas of her brain that coordinate organization and movement.

Wow. When you see your baby lift her head and trunk off the floor for the first time, a brass band should enter from stage left to celebrate the event!

The importance of *intention* must be underscored. All human beings have the hardwiring to physically develop, no matter how much stimulation occurs. In essence, barring any serious neuromuscular conditions, all babies will eventually learn to walk and talk. How organized they become in their everyday performance is another matter.

Bilaterality Emerges

Another mariachi-band moment occurs when your baby brings two hands together voluntarily. You can play "Pat-a-Cake" and hold your baby's hands while clapping them together. This helps your child feel and learn the movement. When your baby claps independently, she has figured out that there are two sides of her body and that they can, indeed, work together.

This hallmarks the beginning of *bilaterality*, an aspect of motor control that is essential to almost all tasks. A tennis player may be right handed and have a one-handed backhand, but ask any tennis pro about proper strokes and he or she will insist that the nondominant hand leads or follows every motion—pointing at the ball, follow-through, etcetera. The nondominant

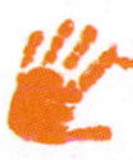

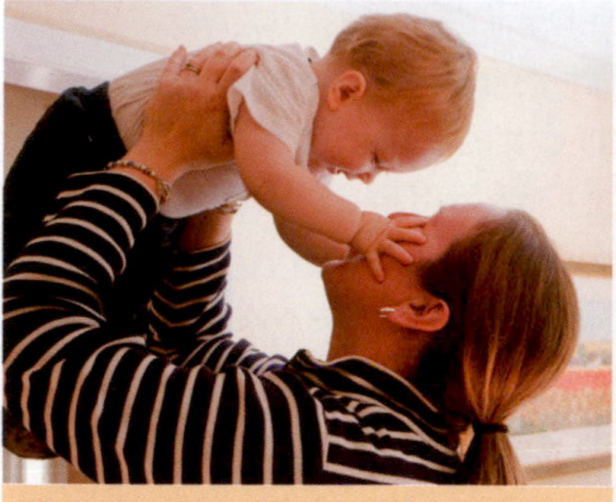

Figure 17. Bilaterality begins! Harrison pats Mommy's face with both hands.

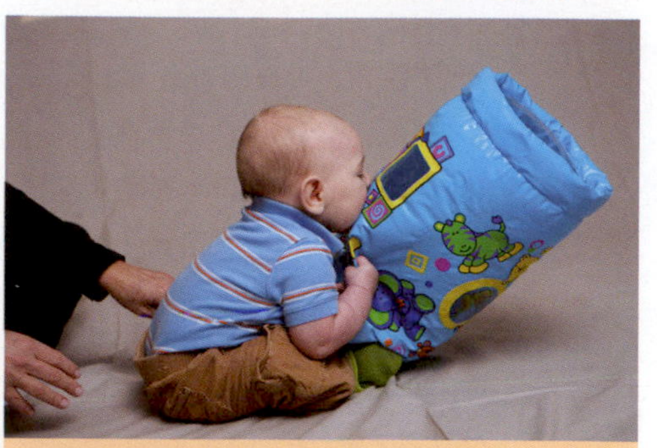

Figure 18. Bobby pulls the toy to his mouth with two hands, demonstrating bilaterality.

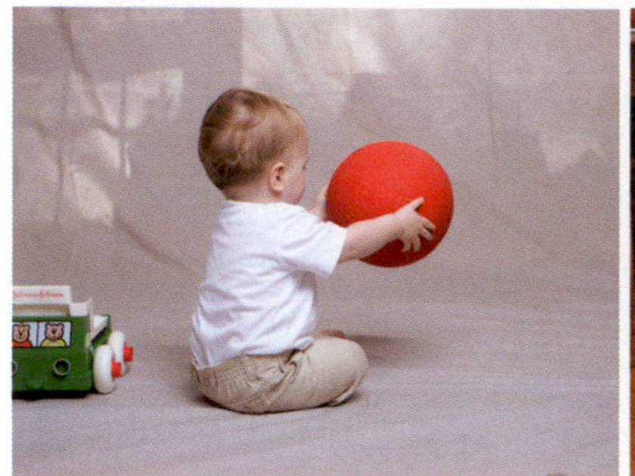

Figure 19. Holding onto a big ball with both hands also demonstrates bilaterality.

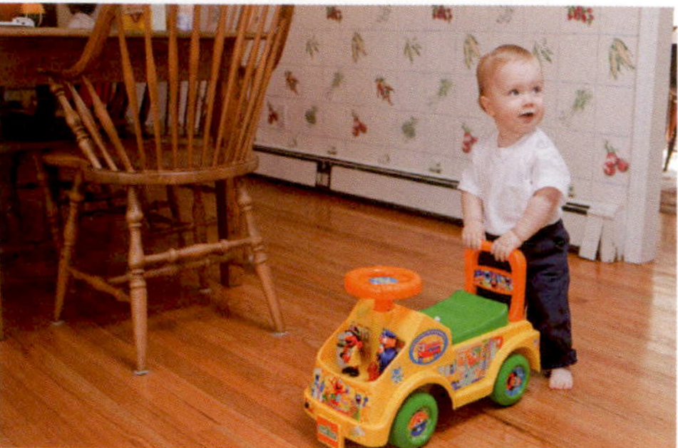

Figure 20. Pushing a toy with two hands.

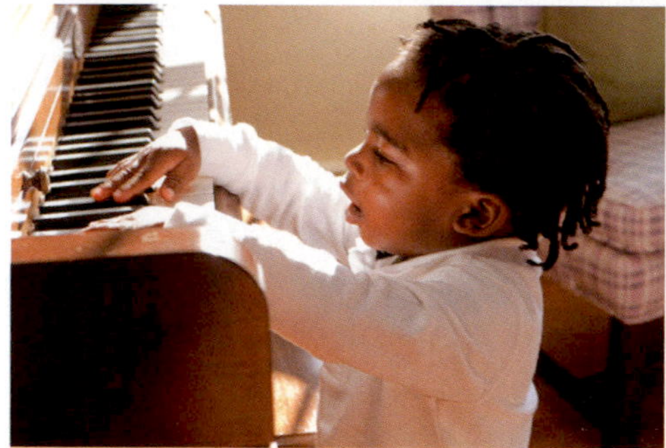

Figure 21. Both hands pound the keys of the piano.

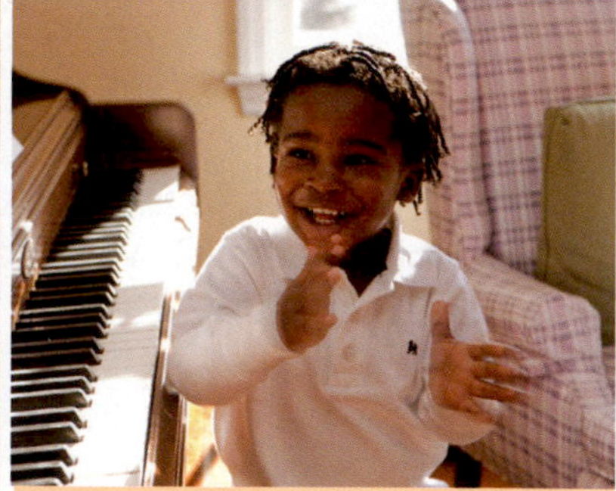

Figure 22. Clapping!

hand assists in almost all tasks. An individual writes with a preferred hand, but without the support of the other hand, the paper shifts on the table and can be very frustrating.

There are several kinds of bilateral activity. The first and easiest

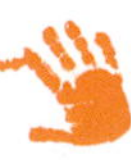

to achieve is when both hands do the same thing. Clapping and patting legs and rolling out play dough with both hands are simple bilateral activities **(Figures 17-22)**. Very early baby games, such as "How big is Susie? Sooo big!" where a baby lifts both arms into the air, help develop rudimentary bilateral skills. Later, a toddler develops bilateral skills in his legs by scooting around on a ride-on toy. Both his feet push off the floor at the same time, making the same motion to move the toy.

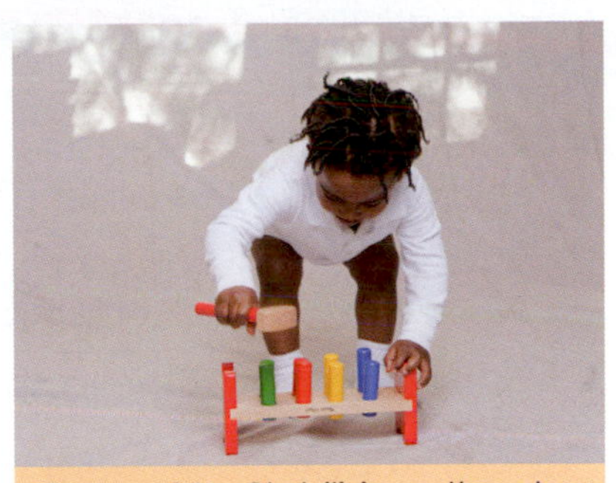

Figure 23. Stabilizing the toy while the other hand bangs is a bilateral reciprocal activity.

Bilateral reciprocal activities occur when each hand or leg has a different job to do **(Figures 23-26)**. This is more complicated and develops after simple bilateral ability is firmly established. With reciprocal activity, each side moves in a different way. Examples Include:

- Pedaling a tricycle: One leg pushes a pedal down while the other leg lifts up.
- Swimming the backstroke: As one arm lifts over the head, the other pulls under the water. There is an alternating motion as the feet kick. (Conversely, the butterfly stroke involves both arms and legs moving exactly the same way, at the same time. While it is a very difficult stroke to do, the butterfly stroke is a *simple bilateral action.*)
- Drumming: Each hand beats the drum individually, typically following a rhythm. (Banging on a drum with both hands at the same time would be a *simple bilateral activity*. Typically, a toddler begins by beating the drum with both hands together, in a static "bang, bang, bang" pattern.)

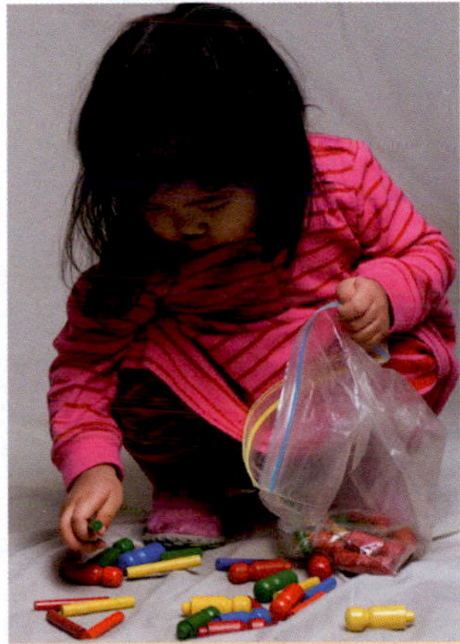

Figure 24. Holding the bag while picking up toys is a bilateral reciprocal task.

Another kind of bilateral reciprocal activity occurs when one hand has a specific task and the other has a different but complimentary job to do.

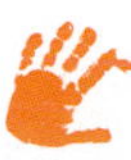

Many activities of daily living require this kind of reciprocal use of both hands:

- Cutting with scissors: The dominant hand manipulates the scissors, while the other hand holds the object to be cut.
- Buttoning: One hand pushes the button through the hole, while the other pulls it through the other side.
- Untwisting lids: One hand holds a jar securely, while the other turns the lid.
- Writing: One hand moves the pencil across the paper, while the other holds the paper still **(Figure 27)**.

With each of these activities, a person needs to feel what the other hand is doing. This requires good touch or tactile discrimination, as well as feeling how the hands and fingers are moving. For instance, with buttoning, first the fingers need to feel the button coming through the hole, then determine the precise moment necessary for the one hand to stop pushing and the other hand to begin pulling. With "advanced buttoning," even more cooperation occurs. Fabric is being pushed and pulled by the fingers not holding the button to ease the movement of the button through the hole.

When a baby begins to use both hands together, the right and left hands mimic each other, doing the same motion. An example would be clapping. When a baby is clapping, a uni-

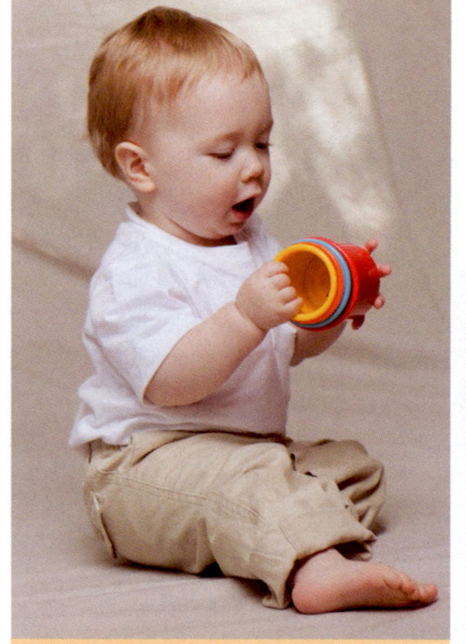

Figure 25. Another bilateral reciprocal activity is pulling toys apart!

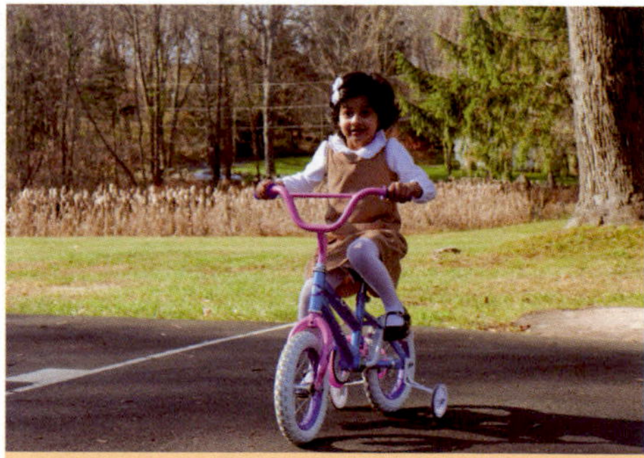

Figure 26. Riding a bicycle is a more complex bilateral reciprocal activity that requires the pushing down of one foot while the other lifts up.

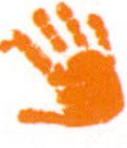

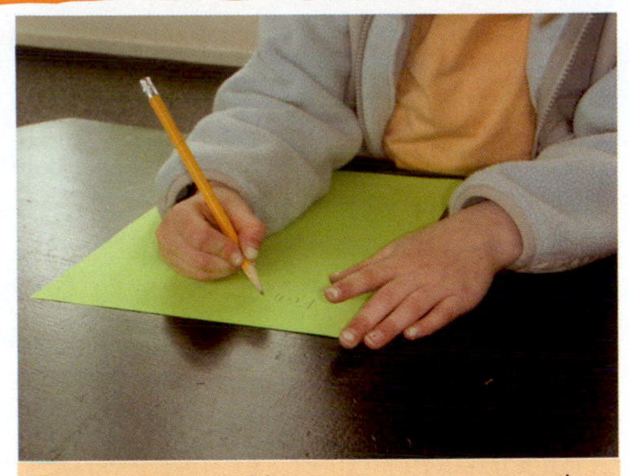

Figure 27. Writing, a more complex bilateral reciprocal endeavor, requires an ability to detect how to hold the paper still as the pencil glides across it, causing the paper to shift.

form message is being sent to both sides of her brain. When the movement occurs, there are places in the nervous system where a crossover or communication of the motion signal occurs. It begins with nerves in the spinal cord. Crossovers continue in the brain, with information traveling from one side of the brain to the other. This is called *interhemispheric communication*. With bilateral movements, the brain receives signals from both sides of the body and transfers the information to the opposite side of the brain. This helps facilitate interhemispheric communication in the brain. Simply stated, the right side of the brain talks to the left side, and vice-versa.

Along with all of the tasks listed previously, there are many basic movements that facilitate the use of both sides of the body, which enhances bilateral development. When a baby pushes up to look around while lying on her tummy, both of her arms are working together. As her legs flex up to push her body toward an object, a coordinated bending and straightening motion of each leg develops. Eventually, reciprocal patterns replace the simple push-pull of scooting, and crawling takes over. We'll talk about crawling, cruising, and walking in depth later in this chapter and in the next. However, it is important to understand that each of these is actually a bilateral activity!

Between the age of 4 months and the time when a baby starts to walk, she begins to roll, push her body up away from the floor, and use the right and left sides of her body in a coordinated way. All of these activities help fire up the organizing parts of her brain. Rolling stimulates her vestibular system. When she pushes up, her proprioceptive system is activated. When she reaches, her kinesthetic system comes into play. While this occurs, her visual system is usually guiding and adding to the motor and sensory experience. When sounds and words are added to the

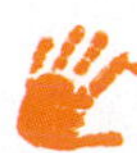

mix, your baby has a very rich set of experiences to organize and act upon.

Early reaching and grasping, stretching her body to obtain toys, rolling over, and lifting her head to look around all provide necessary building blocks for fine-motor and bilateral skills. Each of these amazing accomplishments facilitates further development. Reaching and grasping become more directed and accurate. She learns to bring her hands together to provide touch exploration with both hands. As your child engages in bilateral activity, she uses her hands less frequently to support her trunk. As a result, her body learns to maintain balance without the support of her arms. Independent sitting soon follows.

Recommended Activities

Here are some activities to stimulate bilaterality in your newborn and growing infant:

- Gently move her hands and arms together in various motions.
- Play games such a "How big is (baby)...so big!" and "Pat-a-Cake."
- Provide opportunities to grasp objects of various shapes and sizes.
- Provide opportunities to grasp large objects (ones that require the use of both hands) with assistance.
- Encourage her to use both hands simultaneously, such as banging objects together.
- During diaper changes, move her legs together, back and forth and side to side.
- While lifting her up and down, tap her feet on a solid surface (as in a dance).
- When she's splashing water in the tub, encourage her to use both hands and/or legs at the same time.

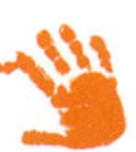

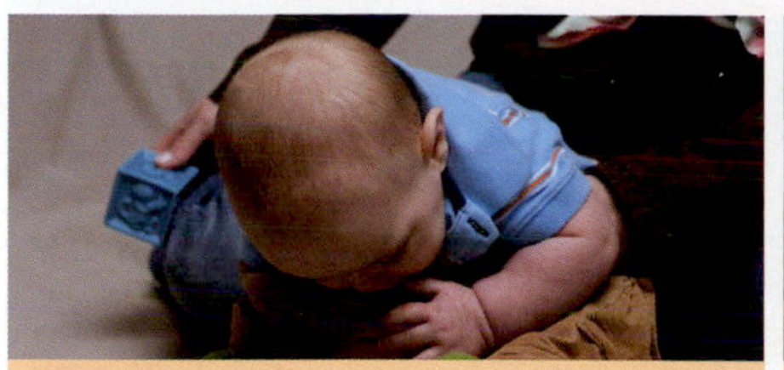

Figure 28. On the road to sitting. Curled up like a pretzel, Bobby doesn't yet have the trunk strength to sit upright on his own.

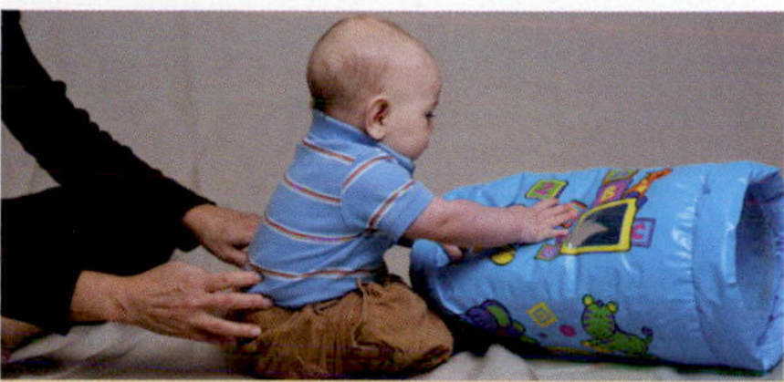

Figure 29. With a little support provided to his hips and lower back, Bobby is able to sit in an erect position.

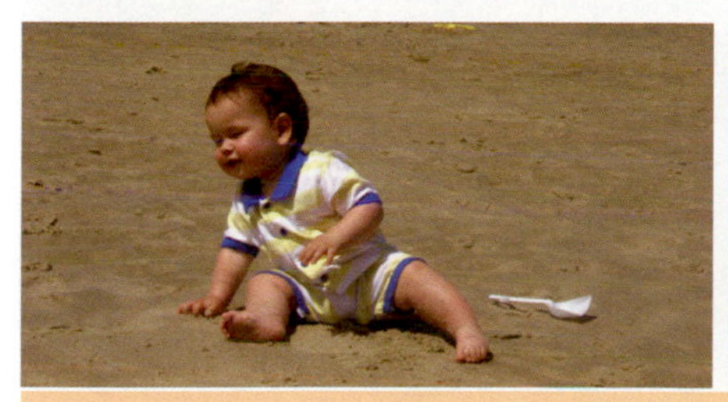

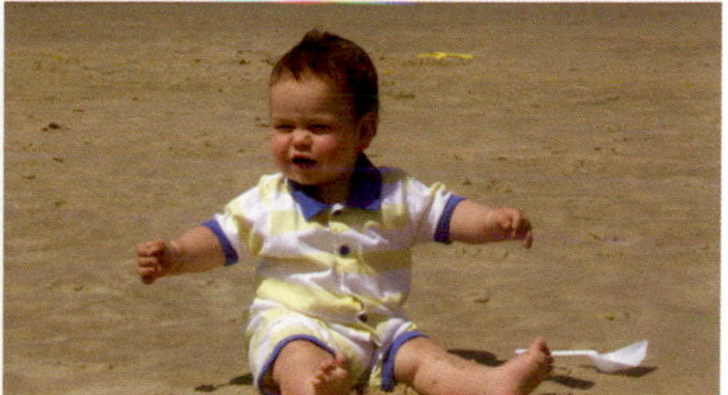

Figure 30. (a) and **(b)** Early attempts at independent sitting require help from the arms.

Independent Sitting

Most parents recognize the importance of independent sitting. Some babies begin the journey to independent sitting as early as 4 to 6 months. Others need more time. When a baby sits with a slumped or rounded back position and hands firmly planted on the floor for support, his little body is saying it is not strong enough to sit upright and alone **(Figures 28-30)**.

Along with lots of "tummy time," engage your child in supported sitting games. Place your baby in your lap, gently bouncing and shifting him from side to side so a slight tilt of his body and head occurs. This activates his trunk and neck muscles to keep his body upright. Leaning your child backward just to the point before his head falls back and then returning him to an upright position can become a fun game, especially when affectionate nose nuzzles or kisses are involved **(Figures 31 and 32)**.

Encourage reaching when your child is in supported sitting positions. This helps activate stomach, side, and back muscles in his trunk. As these muscles develop, his body becomes strong and can maintain an upright position **(Figure 33)**.

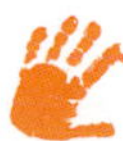

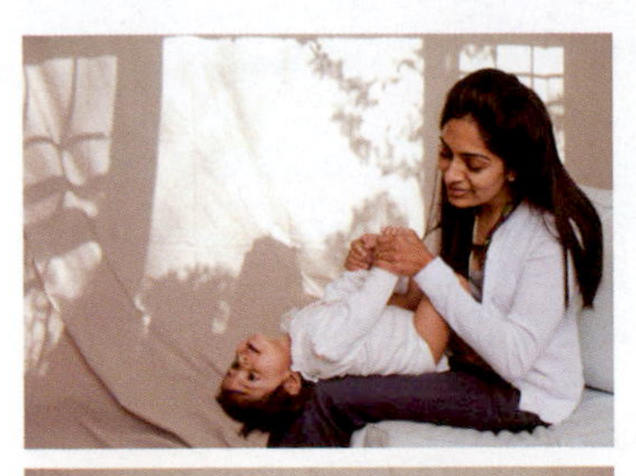

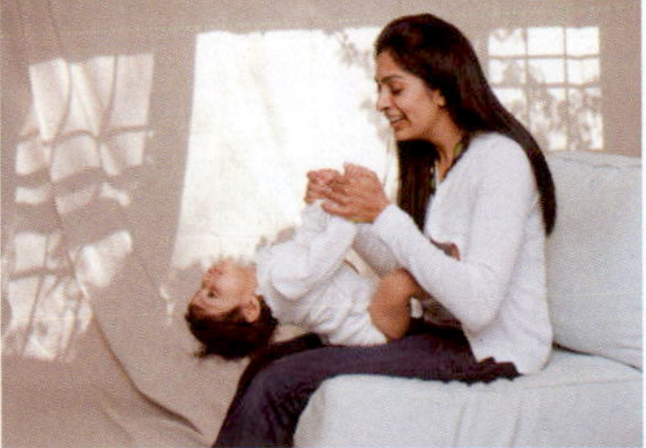

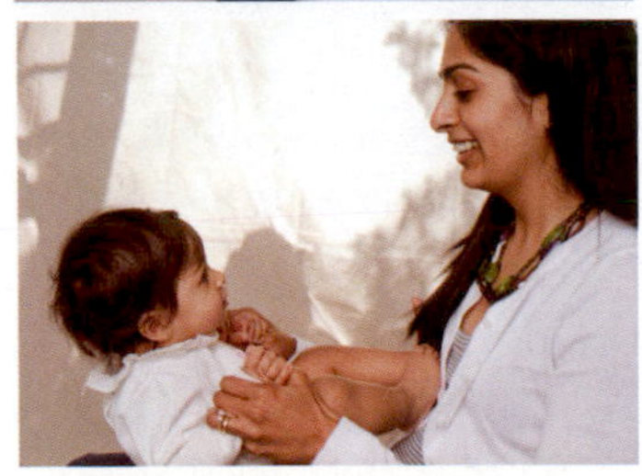

Figure 31. (a) Vedha is slowly lowered backward. **(b)** With Mom's help, she sits back up. **(c)** Note the eye contact. What a fun way to have a caregiver's undivided attention!

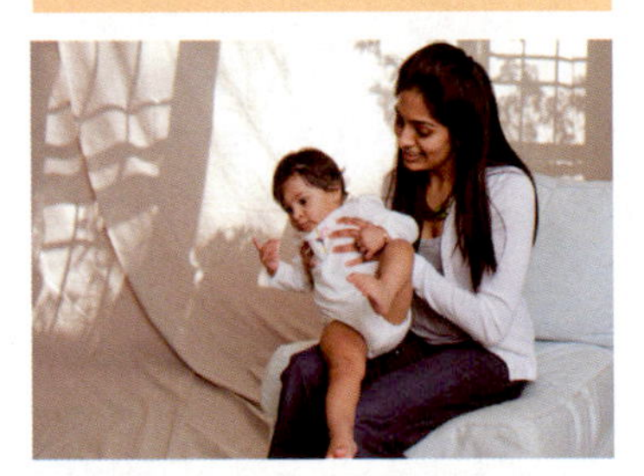

Figure 32. Sideways-tipping challenges a baby's body with new sensations that improve equilibrium reactions, as well as trunk strength.

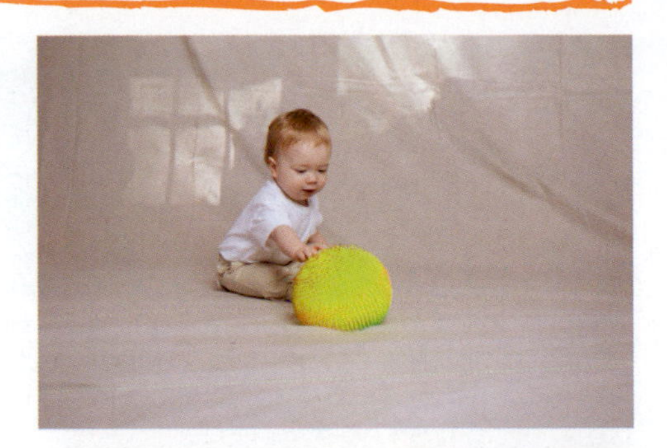

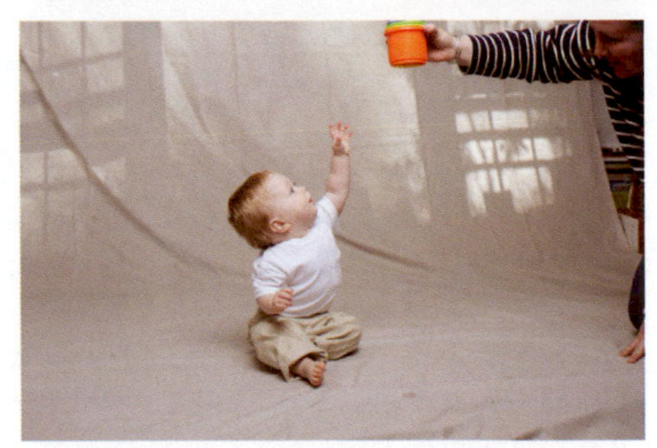

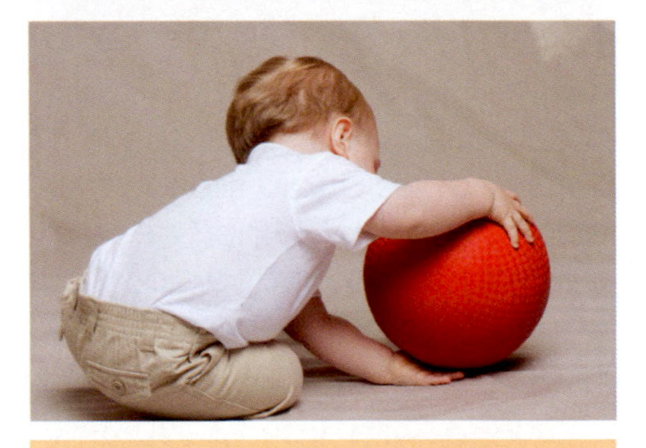

Figure 33. (a) Balance challenges to strengthen independent sitting. Encourage your child to reach to the right and left sides of his body, as well as above his head. **(b)** Reaching activities like these strengthen the muscles in the trunk. **(c)** Encourage the child to reach with both hands, as this requires more trunk work. Large, inflatable beach balls work well for this activity. Younger children can also participate if you sit on the floor and position them between your legs for added support.

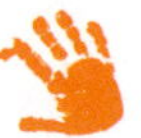

Once your child masters independent sitting, many wonderful things occur. His arms are free to explore, and both hands can manipulate objects and reach new distances to obtain toys. This extended reaching further strengthens his trunk muscles, especially side or lateral muscles, as they stretch to the limit and then pull his body back up to a sitting position.

This "extreme reaching" initiates great things. Good balance is required to prevent falling. Equilibrium reactions and postural adjusting are "tools" used by your baby to figure out how to move his body to maintain his center of gravity and prevent flopping over. The more often his body is challenged through reaching, the "sharper" these tools become.

Eventually, this "extended reaching" pulls your baby over into an approximated four-point (all fours) position. This is another "Aha" moment! The inadvertent transition to all fours leads to the ability to move from a sitting position to a crawling position. The potential to take off, to move without the assistance of an adult, dawns on the child for the first time.

Recommended Activities

Keep in mind that being patient as a parent is pivotal, as sitting is a developmental process. The timeline of when your child's trunk muscles grow strong enough for independent sitting varies.

- Provide supported sitting opportunities in your lap, on the floor with cushions, or on a soft surface so falling over will be a pleasurable experience.
- Provide opportunities for your baby to strengthen his trunk muscles, such as tummy play.
- Provide balance challenges while your baby is in a supported sitting position. For example, while sitting on your lap, tip your baby forward, backward, and side to side in a gentle and fun way. Make sure he is well supported, engaged, and enjoying the sensation of tipping. An exercise ball can be substituted to provide more of a challenge. Make sure your baby is well supported. However, your lap provides more opportunity for close interaction, eye contact, and warm touch.

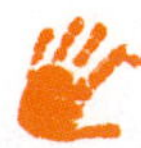

The Case for Crawling

In our bipedal society, functionally speaking, walking trumps all, but in terms of motor development, the importance of crawling overshadows walking. When looking at the contribution to overall motor development, crawling is pivotal.

Four-point, or crawling, movement requires a continual adjustment as the center of gravity changes with each movement of the legs and arms. This requires sophisticated shifts of body positioning and balancing to correspond with the motor sequence. This further enhances dynamic balancing, which began with independent sitting.

The lift and placement of each arm and leg form a complex motor sequence. It is a reciprocal bilateral activity, which is so helpful with brain organization, as reviewed earlier **(Figures 34 and 35)**.

Crawling also works the trunk muscles extensively. Ask any adult who spends several hours crawling around on the floor playing with a baby. The "heavy work" stimulates proprioceptors, which are so important for brain organization.

In addition, crawling requires a slight lateral bend and stretch of the trunk. This strengthens muscles that wrap around from the front of the body to the back. These muscles are used especially when reaching across the midline of the body.

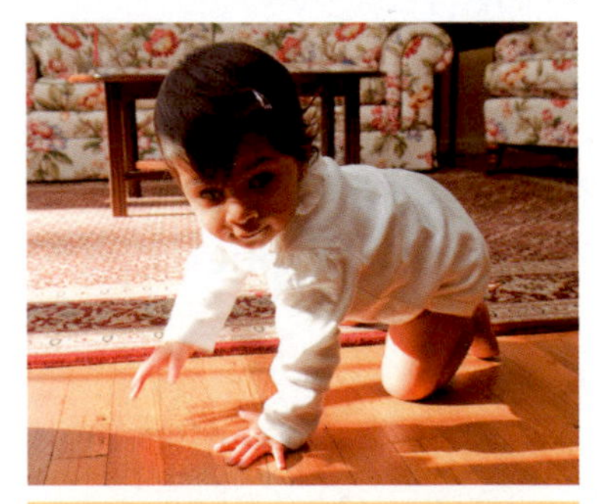

Figure 34. As Vedha crawls, her right hand lifts and reaches as the opposite (contralateral) leg moves forward. As a proficient crawler, the left arm lifts as soon as the right is placed on the floor. The legs follow a similar alternating pattern.

Ease of movement across the midline frees the body up for establishing dominance. Once reaching across the body to obtain an object can be done with ease, the hand wired to dominate will take over most of the refined work as fine-motor skills develop. However, if a child feels insecure about reaching because of a fear of losing his balance or the effort entailed, he will grab objects with the closest hand—the left hand for objects on his left side and the right hand for objects on his right side.

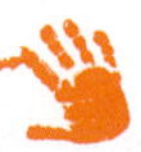

When this happens, delays in developing a dominant hand may occur.

Many of the children who are referred to me have not learned to crawl. When discussing their developmental histories, many of the parents crow that their child was a precocious walker and skipped crawling. To physical and occupational therapists, this is a red herring. When children skip crawling, they miss out on many of the crucial motor underpinnings that bolster strong motor development.

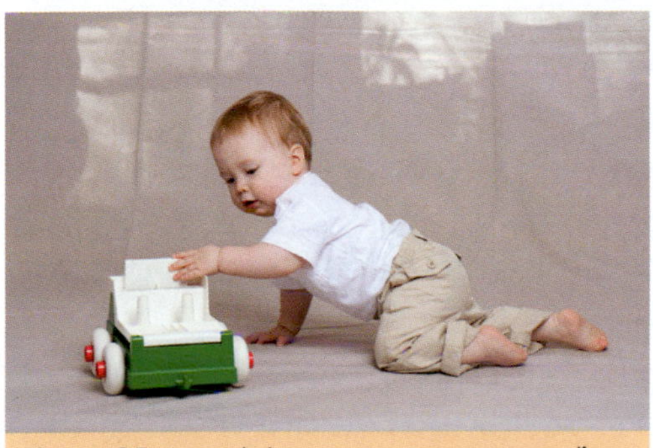

Figure 35. A push toy encourages crawling.

Scooting is often a precursor to crawling. A baby drags his body across the floor by pushing and pulling. For children with weak bodies, this serves as a substitute for crawling. Scooting provides tremendous opportunities for trunk strengthening, activating gravity receptors and other motor organizers. Even after a baby masters crawling, cruising, and walking, scooting is still a terrific movement to incorporate into the play repertoire. An example would be scooting into a "tunnel" made of blankets.

Because crawling is a highly integrated motor task, there are many things that need to develop to be able to crawl.

1. *Strength in the trunk,* especially strong back muscles and stability in the joints
2. *Dynamic balancing,* so that adjustments can be made as the arm is lifted and moves forward
3. The ability to *coordinate several movements in a specific sequence,* as well as *use both sides of the body in a coordinated way*

There is great variability in when and how a child learns to crawl. Here is a typical developmental progression. I have included this to highlight developmental tasks that usually occur along the road to crawling. It should not be used as a cookbook recipe that each child must follow!

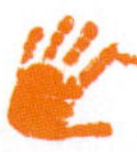

- *Between 4 and 5 months,* a baby pushes his body up, with his shoulders off the floor, while lying on his tummy. His legs may pull up and under his trunk. He may be able to push forward with his knees.
- *Between 6 and 8 months,* sitting stability develops. This strengthens the trunk and hip muscles necessary for crawling. Dynamic balancing begins to develop in his trunk.
- *Between 4 and 8 months,* his legs begin to push his trunk forward. His arms begin to either pull his trunk forward or push his body backward. This is not done in a coordinated fashion yet.
- *Between 6 and 9 months,* a four-point position (on hands and knees) is assumed. Sustained weight-bearing and rocking back and forth occur, but the baby remains stationary. After this is accomplished and endurance increases, the child is ready to reach out and begin to crawl.

I watched with fascination as my son, Ben, got up into a four-point position and executed arduous exercises that led to crawling. For an entire week, he would get up on all fours and rock back and forth many times a day. I eagerly waited for the moment he would move his arms forward and begin to crawl. Sure enough, the day came, and he cautiously moved off the blanket. His twin sister, Kate, who was engaged in her own little tummy-time activities, suddenly shifted her attention to her brother's maiden voyage across the room. Without a moment's hesitation, she got into a quadruped position and followed him. While Ben went through an excruciating process to ready his body for the task of crawling, his sister somehow acquired the necessary strength and ability seemingly without effort, and when her twin introduced the idea of independent movement, she was ready and able to go. The same blanket, same toys, same parenting techniques, and even some of the same genetic material were involved—but each child had a unique way of moving through this important developmental sequence.

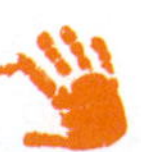

Recommended Activities

Crawling can be facilitated in the following ways:

1. Give your baby plenty of floor time, especially on his stomach.
2. Once your child can sit unsupported, encourage him to reach from side to side to grasp things.
3. Encourage rolling.
4. Engage in weight-bearing games, such as pretending to jump on a caretaker's lap and doing a modified wheelbarrow walk, with the hands walking on the floor while the body is supported.
5. Encourage reaching for and playing with toys while in four-point position (eg, playing with a toy car or ball).

The following are some substitutions for crawling. There is a downside to these substitutions—they do not provide adequate weight-bearing in the joints (fingers, hands, elbows, shoulders, knees, and hips), as crawling does. They also do not challenge your child's balance in a dynamic way, and reciprocal motor sequences are not established.

1. Rolling to his destination—this is effective and facilitates the use of his lateral trunk muscles. It also stimulates vestibular/kinesthetic and proprioceptive input for general neurological organization.
2. Scooting on his tummy—this strengthens his trunk muscles and limbs and provides "heavy work" to stimulate his proprioceptors.
3. Doing the "sit scoot"—this allows him to reach his destination. It primarily strengthens his trunk and hip flexors. There is less development of the back muscles and musculature around his joints with the sit-scoot.

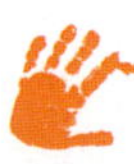

"And Away We Go...!"

The hands continue to strengthen as they grasp objects and bear weight, while pushing the body upward and crawling. At some point, your child figures out how to reach up and grasp the windowsill or couch cushion. Those little hands work along with the developing legs and trunk to push and pull until—voila! Your baby pulls himself up to stand. Another amazing moment!

Imagine the possibilities confronting your new little human being. Suddenly the vista opens up. From a standing position, your child can scan the entire room. Unencumbered by someone's arms or a restrictive device, such as a walker, this miniature individual experiences the thrill and/or terror of freedom for the first time. Your child's personality will come into play here—will she decide to cover more territory and immediately start cruising? Or perhaps the experience seems overwhelming, so she plops down to try again another day.

Once your baby has pulled herself up to a standing position, sooner or later, she will make tentative movements sideways while holding onto a supportive surface, such as furniture. This is called *cruising*. Cruising occurs for varying amounts of time, depending on the child and the environment.

If cruising leads to everything desired in the environment, the motivation to let go may not occur just yet. The child's personality also contributes. The determination and need for independence plays a big part. How ready your child's body is, physically, plays an even bigger role. Are the equilibrium reactions and postural adjusting that are needed to maintain balance present? Does your child have confidence that if a fall occurs, his arms will reach out to protect him? Do his legs move freely from his trunk? Do his eyes guide his body with each attempted stride? Is there an audience waiting to adore your amazing little human being?

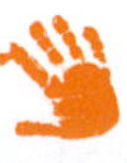

Recommended Activities

Position toys and other objects of interest just beyond reach, so your baby needs to move a little to be able to see or reach for them. Make sure it is a manageable stretch. The objective is to provide a fun challenge, not an impossible mission. A frustrated baby will eventually quit!

Encourage your baby to use both sides of his body whenever possible, such as clapping his hands and moving his legs together in a reciprocal and rhythmic way. When he's grasping toys in an attempt to bring them to the center of his body, assist him so that both hands can explore, manipulate, and hold the objects.

Your baby's arousal level can be enhanced by providing movement and specific tactile input. Light touch, such as tickling, will increase his arousal level. However, care must be taken not to overexcite him, as this state can lead to disorganization, discomfort, irritability, and an inability to focus and engage positively with his surroundings. Swaddling or wrapping him tightly in blankets can help soothe and relax him if he's overly excited. Experiment with rocking, bouncing, and swinging to determine what excites and/or relaxes him.

Assess your baby's surrounding environment:

1. Is it safe to move around?
2. Is it too loud? Too quiet?
3. Is the room visually distracting, or is it uninteresting?
4. Is everything instantly available, or does your child need to plan and work a little to obtain objects?
5. Varying your baby's toys regularly, rather than having all the toys displayed, creates a sense of novelty and increased interest.
6. Is there room to move around and play on the floor?
7. Is your baby dressed in comfortable clothing that allows for freedom of movement? (While absolutely adorable, those crinoline dresses and double-breasted suits restrict movement and do not provide much in the way of comfort.)

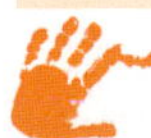

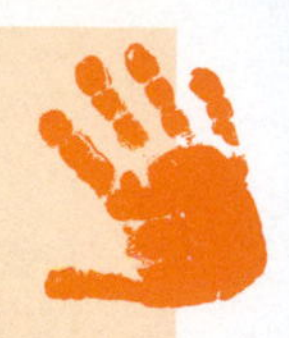

Assess your baby's level of human contact:

- Do you or your baby's caretaker instantly anticipate and satisfy every desire the baby has?
- Is your child left alone for long periods of time?
- Does your child experience human interaction frequently during waking periods, and do these interactions begin with eye contact?

Interaction between you and your baby (or your caretaker and your baby) should coordinate with your baby's arousal state: When he's in an active alert state, motor play with accompanying cheerful banter and attention will bring enjoyment and growth to all.

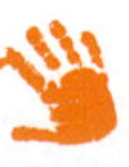

Chapter 3

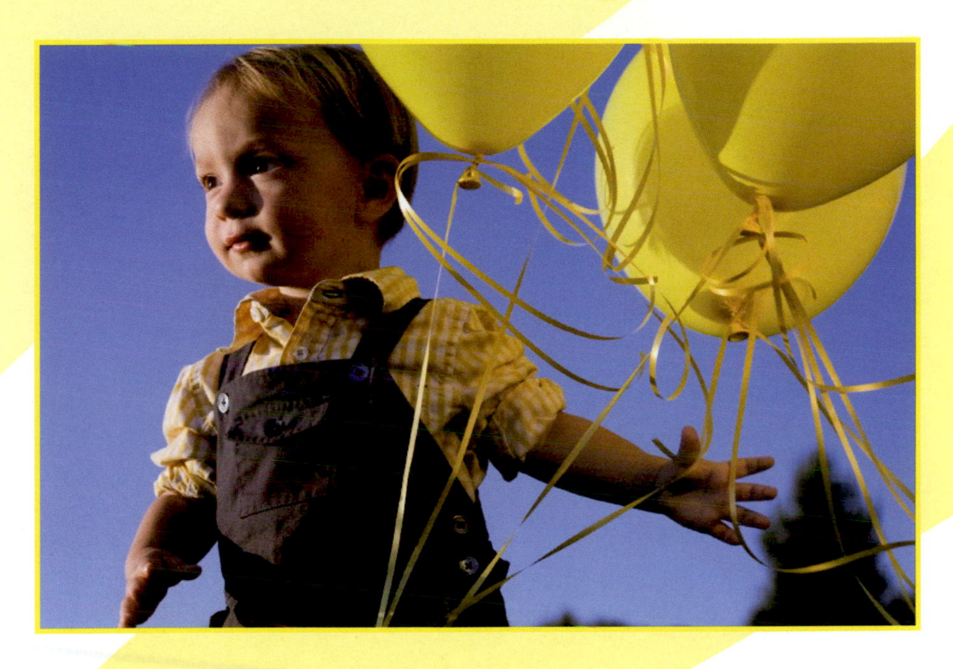

The Road to Walking— The First Year and Beyond

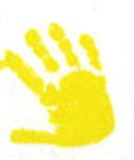

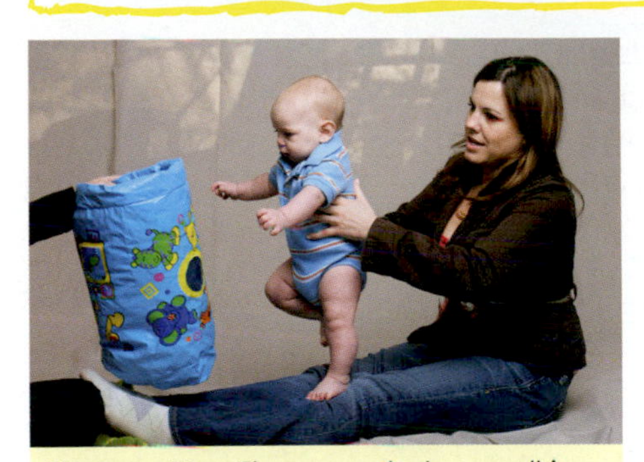

Figure 36. The road to walking. Gradually, Bobby learns to bear more weight on each leg.

Our friend Ashley, from chapter 1, was a sweet and very compliant child, for the most part. But when she first learned to walk, she struck terror into her mother's heart and anyone else who witnessed her hurtling across a parking lot. She was so fixated on the challenge of walking that she would let go of her mom's hand and charge forward in a headlong way, oblivious of anything in her path. Crossing the parking lot felt like a life-and-death struggle for Ashley.

As mentioned earlier, when I began to work with Ashley, she had just learned to walk. Her gait was broad, and her movements lacked the smooth motion necessary to walk in a safe way. She lurched forward in straight lines, accelerating as she moved. Ashley's mother was terrified to watch her careen across a room, especially in public places like grocery stores. Ashley was unaware of anything obstructing her path, and if stairs, shopping carts, or other objects got in her way, she paid no attention. She was clearly missing many of the sensorimotor fundamentals necessary for independent walking.

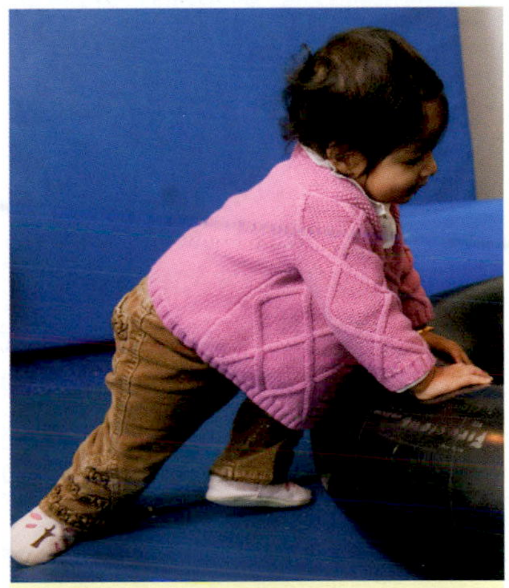

Figure 37. Vedha experiments with partially standing on her own.

Let's discuss these fundamentals in detail. Once your baby gets up on two legs, the many components necessary to become a competent walker, such as *dynamic balancing, grading and control of movement,* and *motor sequencing,* develop over time and with practice. As these improve, proficiency in walking increases.

Getting up and down from the floor, picking up toys, walking in new directions, changing speed, and pulling and carrying toys

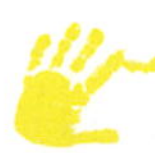

all require additional demands. Finally, as these skills develop, your child will seek new challenges, such as climbing stairs, hopping, kicking balls, and running.

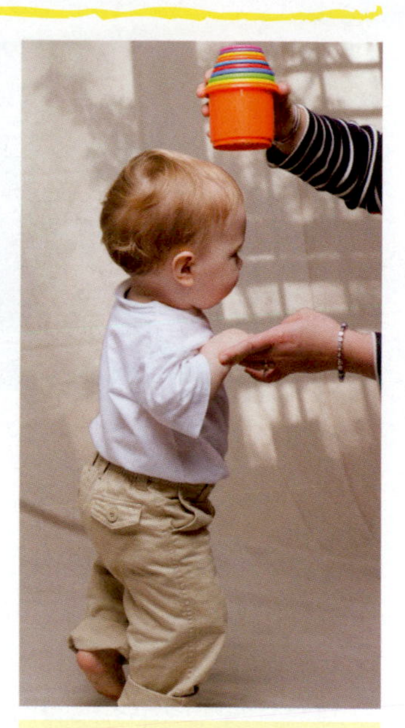

Figure 38. Harrison receives a little help from his mom.

Here's what typically occurs and what must be solidly in place before your child is ready to lift one foot in front of the other and let go:

1. While fully supported, your child will stand on his feet briefly, such as while jumping up and down on someone's lap.
2. Still fully supported, your child will stand for longer periods on the floor. He may practice lifting one leg up, thereby shifting all his weight to his other leg. Movement forward does not occur yet.
3. As his endurance builds, your toddler can be guided in forward movements while holding onto both of your hands. This allows for practice in the "lift-and-place" motion of the legs.
4. Over the next few months, his legs get stronger and his stepping pattern improves. Activities such as pulling up to standing and cruising help strengthen the precursors to independent walking **(Figures 36-38)**.

As his little legs get stronger, his body awareness of how his limbs are positioned and move improves. Besides the "standing readiness" activities listed previously, many other activities help facilitate his readiness for walking. Remember when he was younger, and he discovered his feet? He took delight in playing with them as if they were toys. Gradually, control of the movement in his legs occurs. At first, it begins as random, thrashing movements. Slowly, the movements become more coordinated. Singing little nursery rhymes while moving his legs to the beat of a rhyme during bath time and while changing his diaper heighten his awareness of how his legs can move. Duplicating these simple rhythms and sequences helps facilitate the development of coordinated movement in his

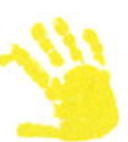

little limbs. Over time, these movements in his legs segue into intentional movement while he's sitting and eventually while he's in standing positions. The complexity of the movements changes from random to simple to coordinated. The timing of motor sequences improves.

The diaper-changing dance sessions, the bath-time splashing, and the rocking back and forth in four-point position all help your baby feel and learn to move his legs in an effective way. As ownership of his lower extremities develops, a sense of control and an ability to direct the movement increase. This leads the way to "cruising" expeditions.

When my first son, Chris, was 9 months old, we joined a playgroup. Each week, we visited someone else's home to play and share in new parenting experiences. Every home we visited could have been photographed for *House Beautiful* magazine. I lamented the day they would all arrive at our house! "Graduate-school furnishings" still dominated our décor, and the early 1970s multicolored shag carpet had yet to be replaced. As I apologized for the state of my humble abode, my friends all exclaimed how lucky I was to have such a baby-friendly environment. They all had to go to great lengths to baby-proof their homes, while I, lucky individual that I was, already had a baby-friendly environment in place. I appreciated their graciousness, and upon reflection, they were actually quite accurate. The incredibly thick pile of the carpet made falling a tolerable experience. The low corduroy convertible sleeper couch was especially easy for my son to hold onto when pulling himself up to stand. Chris was able to cruise from couch to windowsill to overstuffed easy chair and beyond with little effort.

When cruising, your baby can explore the world from the height of 2-3 feet above the ground, rather than only 12 inches. He is able to focus on the movement of each leg. As he gets comfortable with standing while holding onto a support, such as a couch, he lifts his leg and moves it sideways. Initially, both arms lead and a leg follows, with full support provided by holding on. Eventually, a more sophisticated motor sequence develops; a hand-over-hand motion occurs while one leg leads, and the other leg bears the full weight of the body. As the hand-over-hand and alternating foot pattern develops, a rhythmic and sequential pattern is established **(Figures 39 and 40)**.

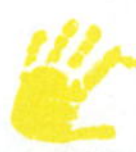

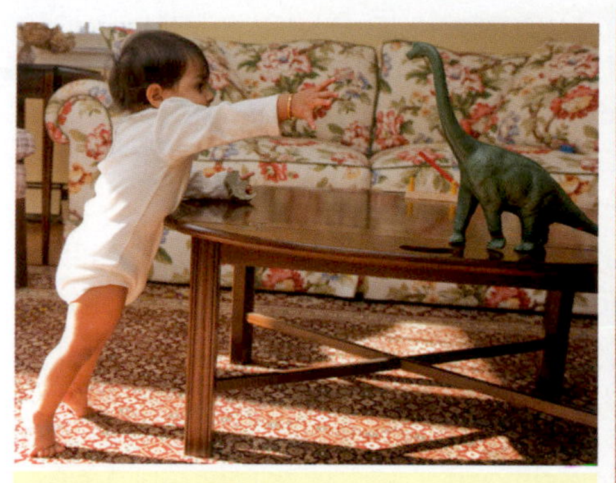

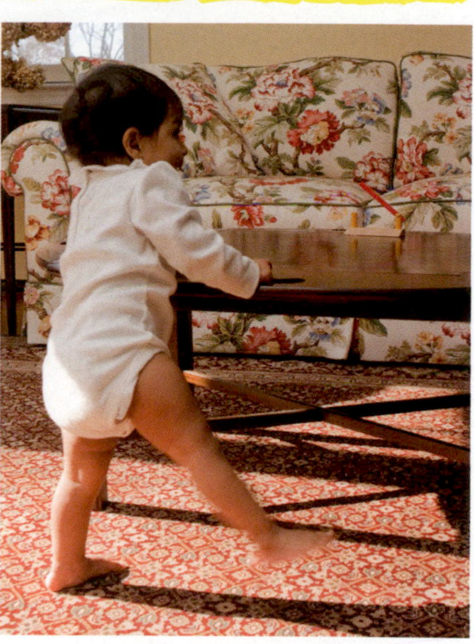

Figure 39. (a) Cruising! Vedha has pulled up to standing, but she's still unable to reach the dinosaur. **(b)** She grabs the table with two hands and begins to move her legs. Note the sideways motion, or gait pattern.

The cruiser might be perfectly content to explore in this manner for quite some time. With enough "cruising supports," a considerable bit of territory can be covered! Your baby may develop a route that traverses the entirety of the room, moving from the couch to the windowsill to the hearth, etcetera. As the vistas from this vantage point are a dramatic change from the low view of the crawler, the child finds a new sense of

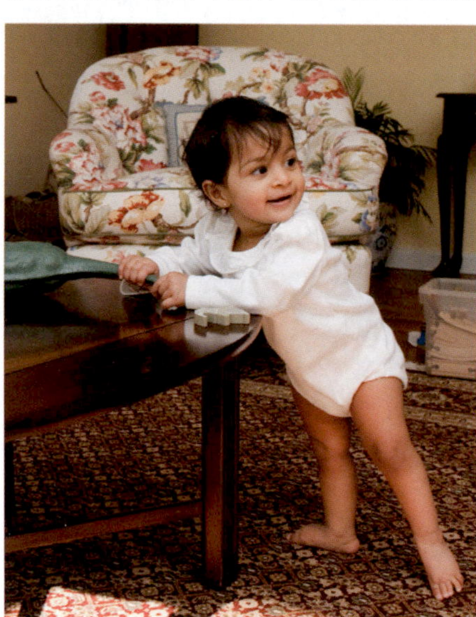

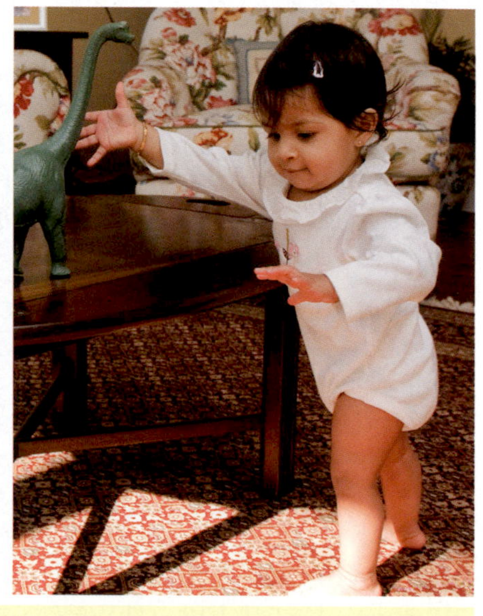

Figure 40. (a) Success! Having reached the dinosaur, Vedha uses her hands to play with the toy as her legs support her. **(b)** Hot stuff! With so much success, Vedha garners the courage to stand alone.

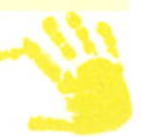

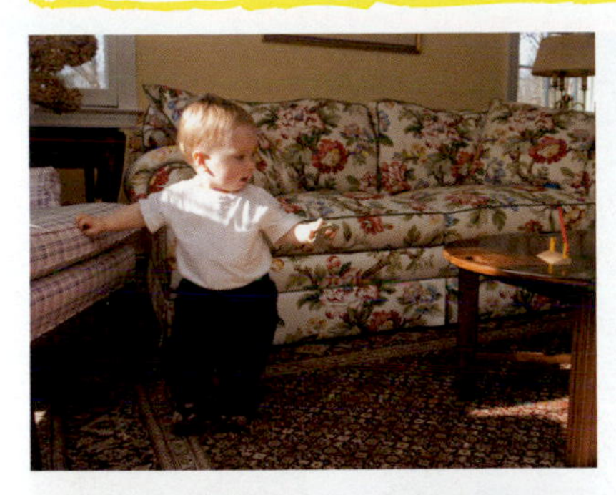

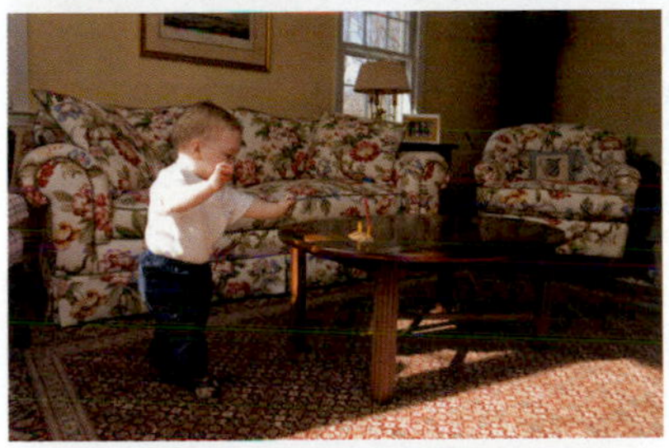

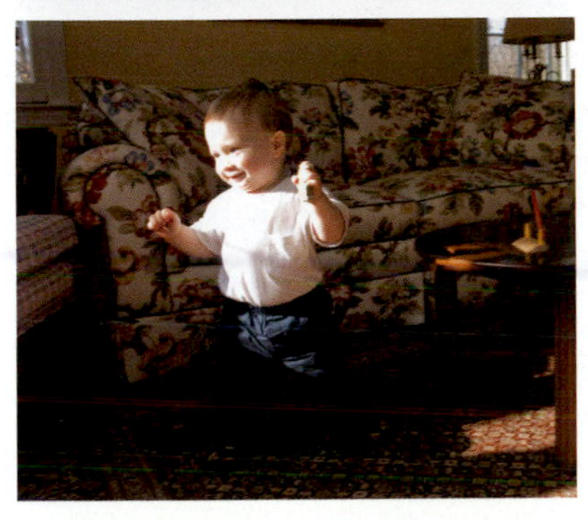

Figure 41. (a) Here and back again! Harrison bridges the gap... **(b) and (c)** Even though he is learning to walk, Harrison still seeks support as he attempts to change directions, carry toys, and start to walk with intent.

freedom and autonomy. Along with a new visual field, objects seen from afar are now an arm's length away. Imagine the possibilities! As your child immerses himself in all the new visual and tactile experiences, his legs continue to strengthen. Balance improves in this new, upright position. Often occurring simultaneously with this cruising period, your baby begins to stand alone, near a support. Slowly, his endurance builds, along with his confidence.

At some point, your child may tire of the cruising circuit and desire a change of venue. Changing routes may lead to pathways with less support available. A gap presents itself, and your cruiser needs to cross over. One hand remains in contact with a support, while his body and legs lunge forward to reach the other side. This may be practiced frequently. Once his confidence, strength, and balance solidify, your baby is ready to take "the first big step!" **(Figure 41)**.

Sometime between 12 and 18 months, your child is ready to let go. Some children wait for a large group, wanting the avid attention of a crowd to take their first steps. Some, on the other hand, choose a quiet moment with just Mom and Dad to cheer them on. Having that adoring adult nearby to validate their big moment really underscores the significance of this outstanding achievement!

Welcome to the world of bipeds! Those first teeter-tottering

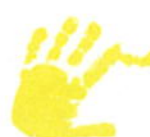

steps lead to a whole new realm of forward motion. Steps are generally taken in a straight line across the room. Then the child plops down and needs a rest. Endurance builds with practice. The task of walking has begun, but there is much work to be done. The toddler must learn the skill of stop-and-go, turning right and left, slowing down, speeding up, bending down, and getting back up. PHEW!

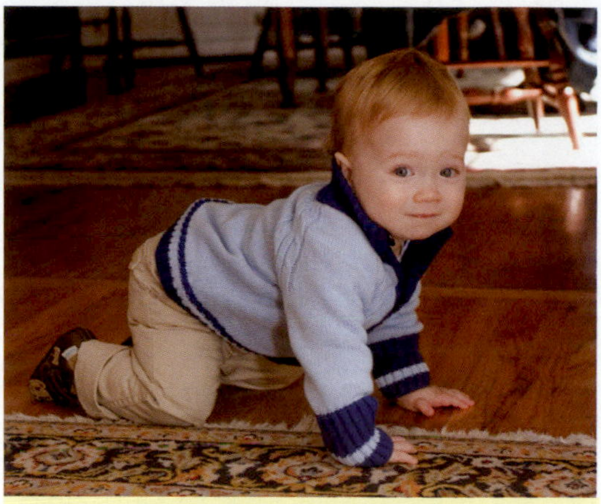

Figure 42. Crawling should be encouraged, even after a child has learned to walk. Harrison is a neophyte walker, but he still enjoys playing on all fours every now and again.

While toddlers are thrilled by their accomplishment, the preferred mode of transportation remains crawling for quite some time. This is a familiar, tried-and-true mode of getting around. When crawling, distance to the floor is minuscule, minimizing the risk of a painful fall. The work of crawling reinforces the feeling of how the body moves and continues to strengthen the very muscles necessary to aid in walking. By the time a toddler begins walking, he has mastered crawling and can reach destinations at breakneck speeds, while walking requires considerable care and courage.

Once your child assumes the biped position, many parents encourage walking exclusively, as though a page has been turned and a new chapter in child development makes the previous one obsolete. Encouraging your child to continue crawling allows him the time and space to build the motor confidence necessary to take future steps independently **(Figure 42)**.

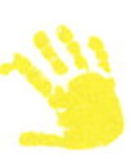

Recommended Activities

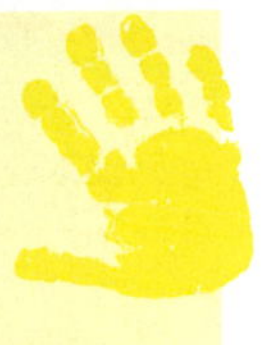

Paradoxically, time spent crawling and playing on his tummy and back helps your child to build the underlying motor control that facilitates walking.

- Provide a safe environment that encourages exploration in independent sitting, crawling, and cruising.
- Consider the placement of cushions and carpets, as well as safe, low, and well-supported furniture that will bear weight and not tip over while your baby engages in cruising.
- Keep safe, interesting objects around for your cruiser to explore, and put away anything breakable.
- For early walking attempts, having bare feet provides more information and the most stable contact with the floor. Socks cause slipping, and shoes are cumbersome at this stage.
- Clear an area for your child to move around in and provide adequate supervision while letting your toddler ramble alone.
- Allow your child to explore his limits and build his endurance at a comfortable pace; provide opportunities to toddle and take sitting and crawling breaks.

Tools of the Walker

As mentioned previously, there are many tasks required beyond putting one foot in front of another and lurching forward into the arms of a welcoming caretaker. Walking requires these key ingredients:

1. Grading of movement
2. Motor sequencing
3. Dynamic balancing

Without these underlying components in place, walking will remain stiff and uncoordinated. Movement on the playground and later on in the classroom might be clumsy or tentative. The child may lack confidence when moving around in busy environments, which ultimately impedes full engagement in play with peers.

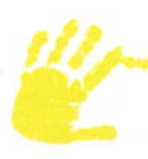

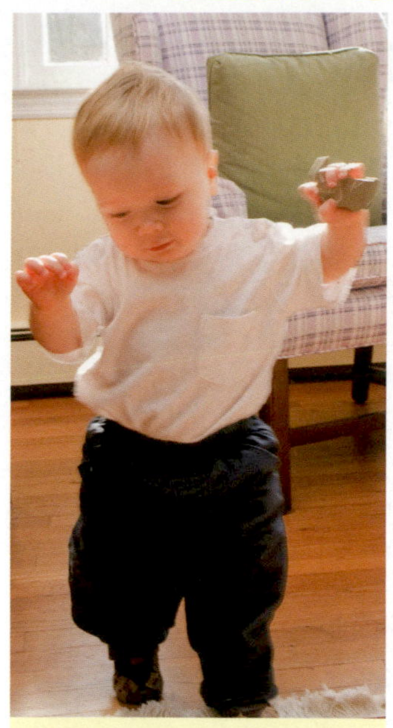

Figure 43. The maturing gait. Early walking requires the use of both arms for balancing, much as a tight-rope walker uses a pole for balance.

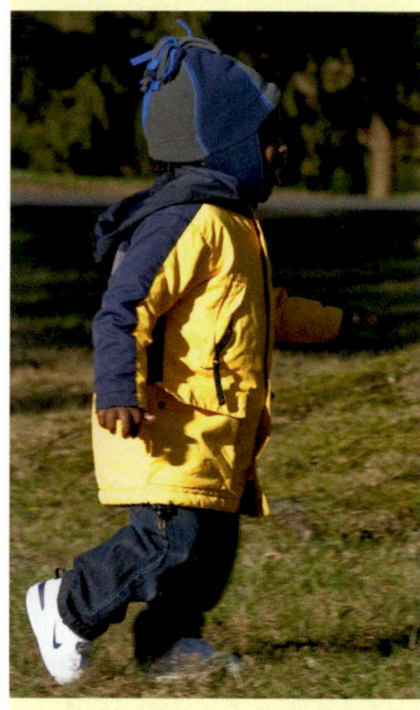

Figure 44. As the gait matures, the arms come down, and a reciprocal arm swinging motion develops.

What exactly is *grading of movement?* This relates to the ability to anticipate the force and speed necessary to accomplish a task. When a toddler reaches for a cup of milk, frequently a miscalculation occurs, and the cup tips over. The child must determine the distance and amount of force required to grasp it successfully.

Grading of movement related to walking takes a subtler form. When toddlers take those first steps, the legs move in an uncoordinated and halting way. With practice, endurance, strength, and balance increase, and the ability to gauge how far to move a leg, and at what speed, improves. This leads to improvements in speed control (slowing down, stopping, and sustaining a consistent speed). When the grading of movement remains underdeveloped, one sees a child who frequently stumbles and crashes into things.

One of the easiest periods of parenting for me occurred soon after my son Chris had learned to walk. The floor plan of our little house included a circular route: The living room opened to the dining room, which connected to the kitchen. The kitchen had a doorway that led back into the living room. Chris would spend long periods of time walking in a halting way around this circuit, over and over again. As he staggered around, he gradually became more proficient in regulating his gait. Over time, he controlled his speed better. The lurching quality of his movements decreased, and he began to stand in an upright position

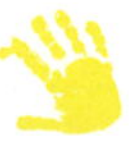

as he moved. He no longer needed to crash into something to stop. Once he mastered all of this, the demands on me as a parent ramped up significantly. Chris had become ready to combine walking with exploring his surroundings!

The series of movements involved in taking a step and then combining these steps into a walking pattern is called a *motor sequence*. Along with how well a toddler "grades" a movement, the way each movement is connected to the next plays a big part in how "fluid" or coordinated walking appears **(Figures 43 and 44)**.

Motor sequences that began to develop early in infancy play a part in the development of the smooth motor patterns required for walking. The "Pat-a-Cake" games, bouncing games in the lap, rocking back and forth in preparation for crawling, and hand-over-hand/stepping patterns of cruising all contribute to the establishment of motor sequences.

These motor sequences help build the neural pathways that link motor centers to motor action. The more often these pathways are used, the more efficient the communication is between the motor centers for coordinating and executing motor action.

The linking of each stepping motion—right foot coordinated with the left—requires timing and accurate execution. With practice, this all comes together. If the motor-sequencing pathways have been firmly established, it is much easier for the child to develop fluid walking patterns.

Think of a musician practicing scales and a ballet dancer working at the barre. The need to activate basic patterns, to make the sequences automatic, is critical to the quality of their performance, no matter how proficient an artist they might be. So it is for the walker: Learning to link simple movements, such as moving the legs back and forth and clapping the hands, helps establish the motor patterns eventually necessary for walking, as well as all advanced athletic endeavors.

Just as those earlier life experiences led to the establishment of fluid motor-sequencing ability, previous balancing activities helped build the stability required to maintain a solid stance when walking. Activities such as reaching for toys while sitting

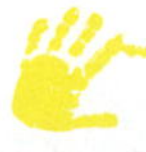

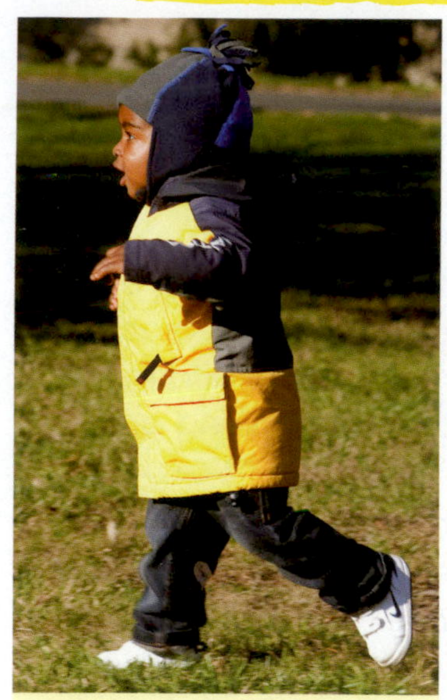

Figure 45. Note that when a toddler runs, his arms come back up into the air. The need for added stability as his speed increases causes this "airplane position" to be used.

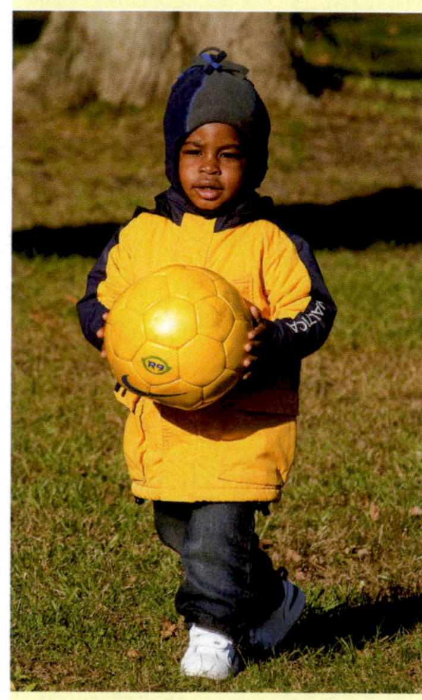

Figure 46. The child can now use both hands to play, since they are no longer required for balancing.

and crawling, maintaining an upright position when bounced or rocked, and early practice with standing and walking all helped develop additional skills for the tool box. *Dynamic balancing* relates to the ability to maintain balance while in motion, whether the movement is inadvertent or intentional. It requires the engagement of many small muscles throughout the body.

Physiologists and trainers have embraced the importance of dynamic movement in exercise programs in recent years. They have added tilt boards and exercise balls to their regimes. Activating the small muscles throughout the trunk for balancing not only burns more calories, it strengthens trunk muscles that have often not been used by adults for many years as a result of sitting behind desks all day. Therefore, the adult body loses its edge in using muscles for dynamic balancing. Sports such as cycling, tennis, and downhill skiing burn more calories than running and basic calisthenics. This is due to the activation of muscle fibers required for the dynamic balancing demands of these sports. Even sports enthusiasts in good condition usually feel new twinges in the muscles of their legs, shoulders, back, and abdominals after a full day of skiing.

Babies, on the other hand, use these muscles constantly when provided with an environment that

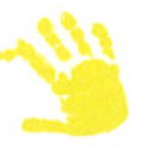

affords ample opportunities to crawl, roll, and generally move around. When engaged in motor activities, babies will reach for toys, going to and beyond the limit of their balancing safety zone. Standing and getting back down repeatedly works many of the muscles so important for dynamic balancing. All of these seemingly simple activities contribute to the essential body responses necessary for the demands of everyday living.

Even earlier in development, when you bounced your baby on your knee with little shifts back and forth, as described in chapter 1, dynamic balancing skills were developing. Each time your baby's little arm swiped at a toy, stretching her torso slightly beyond its comfort zone, the muscles necessary for dynamic balancing were activated.

During her early walking days, your child toddles around, working on coordinating all these components of walking. Her endurance increases, and the tools for proficient walking develop. Smooth motor sequencing, dynamic balance, and grading of the movement of each step improve **(Figures 45 and 46)**.

Soon, your child begins to add new challenges to her repertoire. She works on turning her head to look at something or someone while she's walking. This is not an easy task, as it demands a positional change of the head that shifts her center of gravity slightly and the visual cues she uses for balancing.

Challenges of the Neophyte Walker:

1. Rotating her head and shifting her visual attention while she's walking
2. Carrying a toy
3. Pulling a toy
4. Bending over to pick up a toy
5. Varying her gait: running, backward and side-stepping, twirling, etc

When you're trying to get the attention of your toddler early on in the walking business, your child may appear to ignore your call. This ostensible lack of cooperation relates more to an inability to turn without falling, rather than a growing independence streak. Burgeoning independence will follow later.

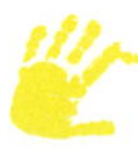

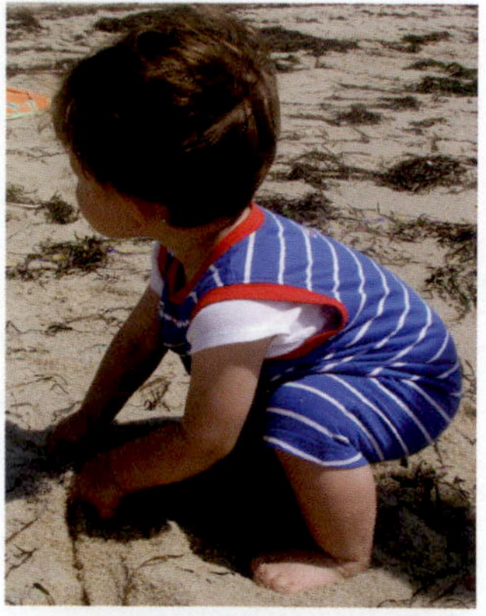

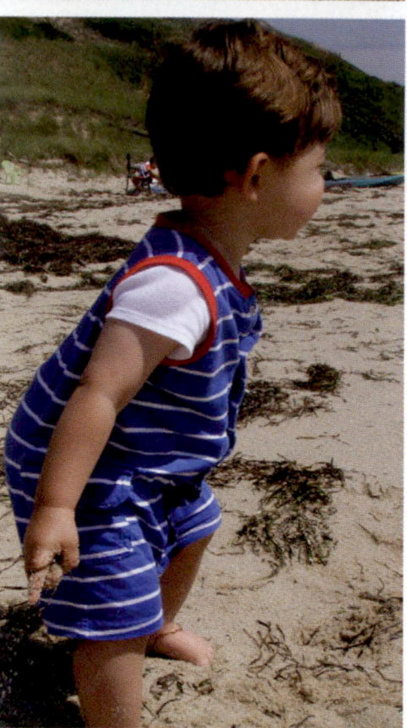

Figure 47. (a) and (b) When a toddler first learns to walk, support from the hands is required to stand up.

Gradually, the range in which your child's head can turn will increase, as her balancing skills improve. Eventually, a full ability to rotate her head and trunk allows your child to look around. Initially, however, she maintains a rigid visual focus, oblivious to surrounding objects and people. She appears to be on one straight track, even if major obstructions litter her path. Over time, she gains competence in her ability to look to the sides, stop, start, and veer in new directions. Sophisticated skills, such as pulling a toy from behind, emerge.

Vision is a very important aspect of balancing. Try standing on one foot and counting to 20. Now repeat this exercise with your eyes closed. It is considerably more difficult. When children begin to increase their range in walking, they move in straight lines for increasing distances. When they reach the end of their safety zone (the distance separating them from their caretaker), they turn around and return along the same path. They do not employ a flexible route. Once their balancing skills improve, their visual field expands, and attention to others in their environment increases. The possibility of moving in new directions also occurs. The straight-line trajectory is replaced by flexible movements. A child can now change directions easily and guide movements with her eyes, as well as her feet.

Carrying a toy becomes another challenge to surmount. Remember that the road to walking began with cruising. Her arms initially clung to an object to help her stay upright while she was moving. Once she let go of that support, her arms still provided her with a balancing counterpoint. Think of the tightrope walker who uses her arms and a pole to assist her in

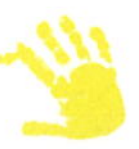

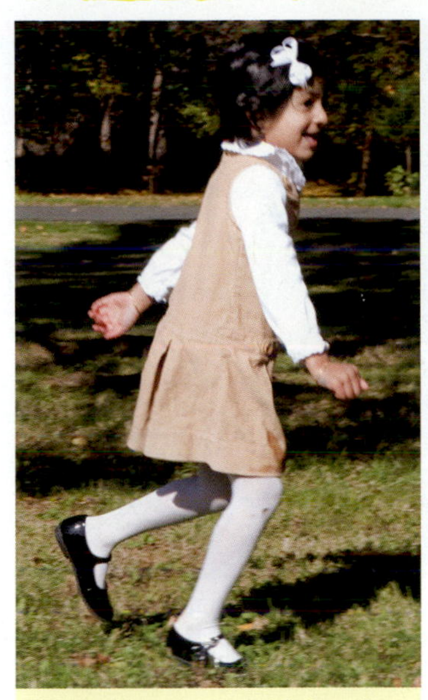

Figure 48. The sophistication of a 4-year-old stride. Aanya comfortably walks and runs, with her arms swaying back and forth in sync with her leg movements.

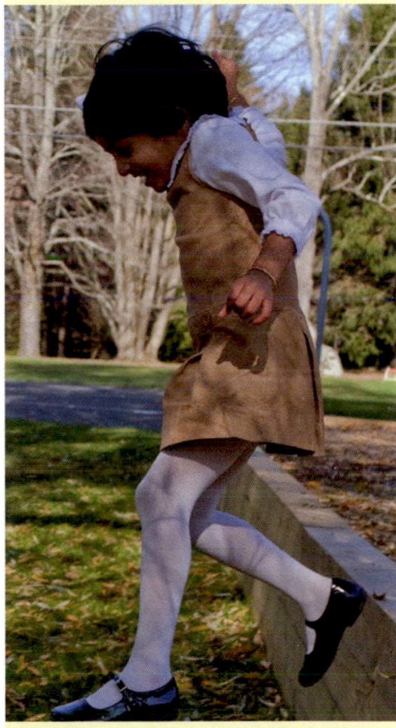

Figure 49. Jumping and climbing become a must.

crossing a wire. When a child brings her hands together to hold onto a toy, it means that the body alone can now do the balancing necessary to maintain an upright position, without the assistance of extended arms.

Along with carrying a toy, picking up a toy off the floor is a major accomplishment. This requires an enormous amount of work. Your child must figure out how to lower her body back onto the floor. She does not want to succumb to falling! Strength in her knees, hip flexors, and trunk is required. Getting back up is equally demanding. Children begin by using their arms, as well as their legs, to push themselves back up into a standing position. Bending over to pick up a toy is a modification of this process, requiring more strength, increased grading of movement, and balance **(Figure 47)**.

Once your child has mastered lowering her body down to the floor, walking around the room or play yard while picking up objects may become an intense and persistent activity. Human development is quite wonderful in this way. As humans work on acquiring and developing a skill, there is an inherent drive to engage in the activity repeatedly until the task is mastered. Having the opportunity to do so is key.

After Chris mastered the art of "walking the circuit" around our house, he worked on a new challenge. He would dump a basket of alphabet blocks on the floor and

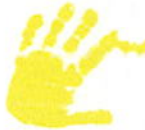

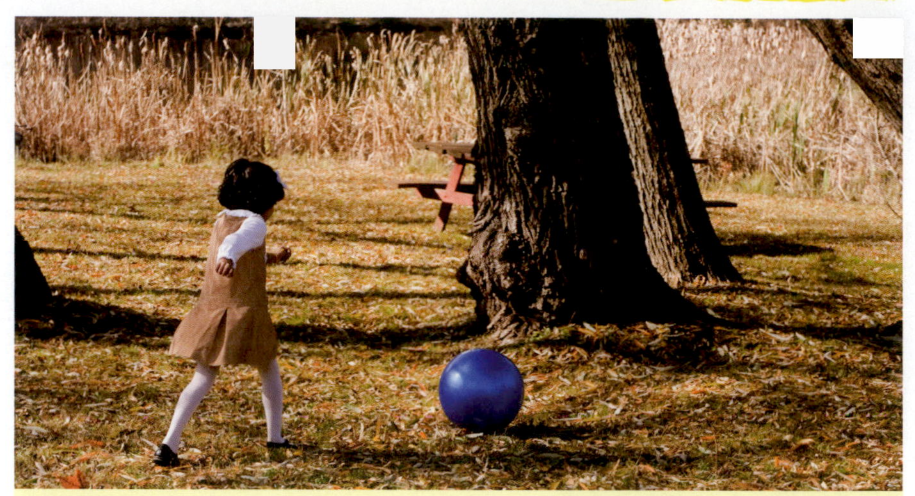

Figure 50. Now Aanya can run and coordinate a kick. Look at how many skills have been integrated: reciprocal arm and leg movements, looking at the ball, regulating speed and direction, and anticipating and planning a kicking movement.

then proceed to stoop down to pick up each one. Immediately upon retrieving all the blocks, he would dump them out again and repeat this performance. After these "workouts," he was delighted to settle down for a story and some rest!

At about 18 to 24 months, a toddler learns to walk in circles and takes great delight in exercising this feat repeatedly. Great pleasure is derived from circling around for admirers over and over again in the middle of the living room. It becomes the star attraction. He also begins to explore moving backward and running. Initially his legs are positioned far apart, much like a drunken sailor. This provides a broad base of support. As the trunk and leg muscles continue to develop, that base narrows, and the child's movement becomes more precise.

I serve as a consultant for several preschools, and children who seem to charge through the classroom, oblivious of any objects or individuals in their paths, are frequently brought to my attention. Dennis was a perfect example. A beautiful child with boundless energy, he loved to play with any and all children in the classroom. Unfortunately, he missed others' cues about maintaining personal space, and his ability to negotiate around the busy classroom was underdeveloped. When he saw a familiar face, he would rush directly toward his friend. En route, Dennis ignored any students playing and

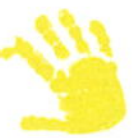

crashed through many a carefully built block structure. As he approached his buddy with open arms, he did not account for the momentum he'd acquired as he hurled himself across the room. As a result, he would crash against his friend, causing them both to topple to the floor.

While a bear hug was intended to cement his friendship and admiration, the opposite usually occurred. Dennis's unintended "victim" was frequently startled by the ferocity of the encounter and cried. Over time, many of the children learned to avoid Dennis. As he entered their space, they would quickly move to protect their block structures and other projects. Often they would avoid contact and yell for Dennis to move away.

Sadly, the unintended result of Dennis's enthusiasm was a lack of friends and eventual social isolation. He became a pariah, not because he was an unfriendly beast, but because he was unable to grade and plan his movement when approaching his friends and negotiating his way around the classroom. He hadn't gained control of the movements necessary for walking—speeding up and slowing down as the situation demanded, changing directions to avoid knocking things over, and using visual cues beyond his one target point to ensure safe movement across the classroom.

An early toddler's focus is acquiring the skill of walking. The greatest pleasure in life revolves around getting from point A to point B, or simply moving back and forth on a random, self-imposed track. Polishing this skill, coupled with the ability to incorporate toys and move in varied ways, preoccupies much of a toddler's waking hours. As seen with Dennis, polishing these skills is very important for future coordination of more complex motor skills. Once competence develops and the new walker becomes more confident, the world awaits, and greater exploration and independence are sought **(Figures 48-50)**.

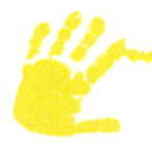

Recommended Activities

- Remember that your toddler will alternate between walking and crawling for quite some time. This is normal and helpful for developing quality walking ability.
- Keep open spaces free of obstructions that may impede or hurt your child. During the early phases of walking, your toddler does not have the ability to negotiate around furniture and other objects.
- Allow your child to get up and down independently. This requires patience on your part, but the effort employed by your toddler is key to the further development of a strong trunk and legs.
- Don't become alarmed if your toddler seems to run away and not come when called. The child is not capable of changing direction, and the stop-go aspect of walking is not established until later in the walking development cycle.
- When genuine fatigue sets in, your toddler will appreciate an "up." Knowing that being held is still an option keeps the challenge of walking in the realm of a positive exercise, rather than a new, overwhelming demand.
- While adult adoration is appreciated and is quite important at the onset of walking, allowing your child quiet exploration time while toddling around the house or yard is important. This provides the child time to process the feeling of walking and become more confident with these abilities. If always distracted by the "cheers," the child has no time to focus on developing walking prowess.
- Set safe parameters and limits, so your child can walk certain distances within the safety net of your (or another adult's) vigilant eyes without feeling a hovering presence. A large aspect of walking independence is precisely that: independence.

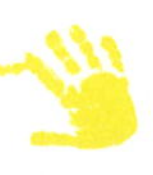

Climbing Stairs

Between 1½ and 2 years old, your toddler will begin to test the limits of his newfound abilities. Lifting a foot off the ground to kick a ball and jumping from a very small height may be attempted. At 2 years of age, your child will enjoy chase games and the opportunity to dance, incorporating whole-body movements such as swinging his arms and legs.

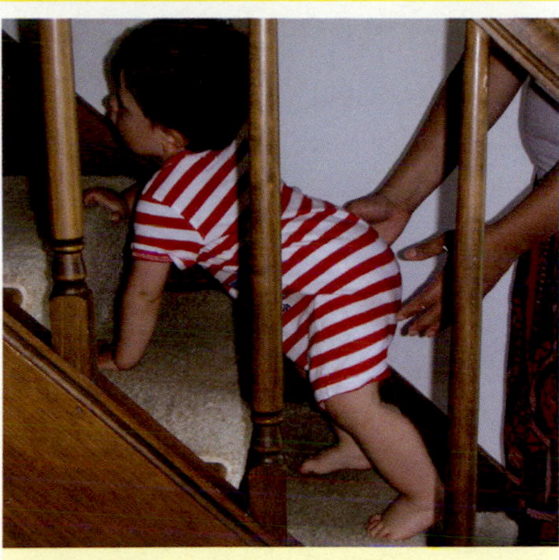

Figure 51. When your baby begins climbing the stairs, your hands should be at the ready!

One of the big fascinations at this time becomes the stairs **(Figure 51)**. Between 12 and 15 months, your baby can crawl up the stairs on his hands and knees. By 18 months, he uses his hands and feet instead of his knees. Both feet rest on the same step before moving on to the next. Going down the stairs comes later. Like getting down from the couch or bed, the same motor pattern is employed for climbing down the stairs. The child backs up to the step and his feet go first, his tummy sliding over it as he lowers himself down.

The level of independence a child displays in climbing stairs varies widely. The normal progression from a modified crawl to walking without any support up and down the steps is as follows.

Typical Progression to Stair-Climbing:

1. Crawling up a step on hands and knees.
2. Using the feet to "step" up, while placing the hands on the steps for added support, with each foot placed on the same step before moving up to the next.
3. Using a railing or the support of an adult, with each foot meeting on the same step before progressing to the next.
4. The need for support diminishes, and an alternating foot pattern (one foot per step) emerges.

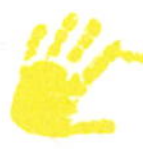

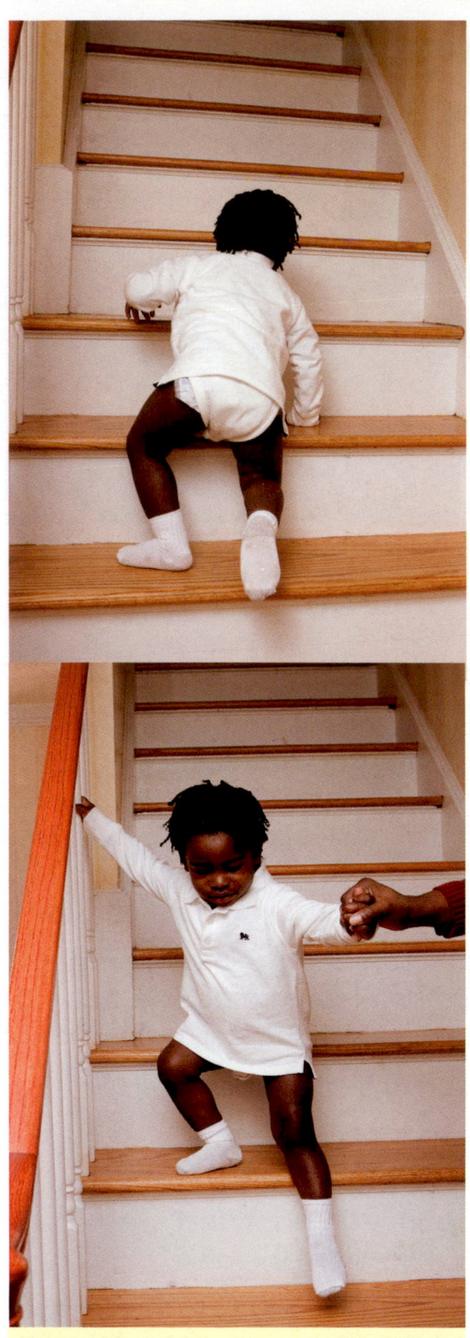

Figure 52. (a) Wayne can now climb up the stairs in a crawling fashion, without help from Mom. **(b)** However, he still needs a helping hand on the way down.

Climbing down stairs follows a similar pattern but lags behind the upward climb **(Figure 52)**. It is scarier to look down and see the distance down the stairs to the bottom. It is also more demanding. Carefully graded movements that require strength and control are necessary to lower each leg to the next step. Most mountain hikers will acknowledge that the climb down is more demanding on the joints and muscles as they carefully lower themselves down the steep trails.

How you assist your child in acquiring safe stair-climbing skills follows the same guidelines as walking. Make sure you're near at hand—in the case of climbing, less than an arm's length away. Waiting patiently and offering some light support without outright holding him will give him confidence and added feedback about where his body is in space—specifically on the stairs. When your toddler is crawl-climbing, providing gentle support at the hips will give him added support on the journey upward. As your climber moves to an upright position, offering firm support to his shoulders reinforces his center of grav-

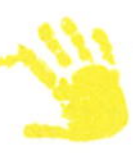

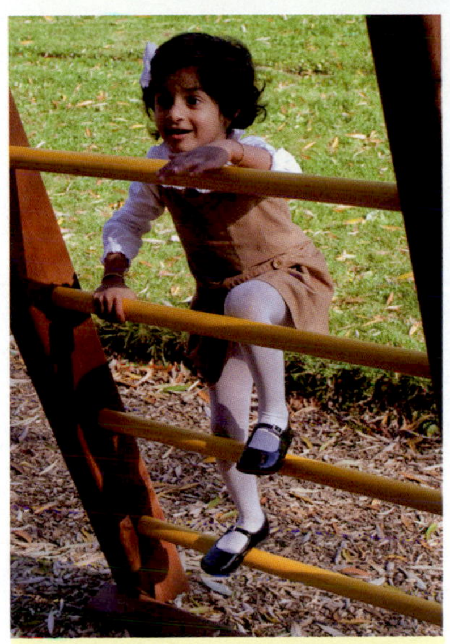

Figure 53. As children grow older, they seek new climbing challenges. Giving them opportunities to try out their growing motor skills is very important. Playground slides, boulders, and stone walls in the park all provide interesting opportunities for climbing.

ity. Providing intermittent and diminishing support should occur as your child gains confidence going up and down the stairs.

Establishing an alternating stepping pattern is quite a bit more difficult and may take a very long time to achieve. It requires nice rotation in the trunk and significantly more developed balancing skills. Playing games that require crossing of the midline, such as swinging a bat and rolling, will help strengthen the muscles necessary to accomplish this **(Figure 53)**. One does not expect a child to accomplish climbing up and down the stairs with alternating feet until about 4 years old.

Recommended Activities

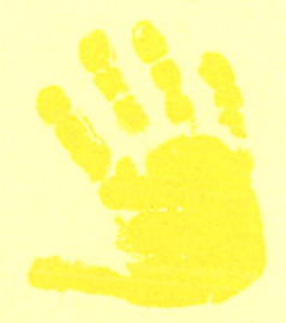

- Provide close supervision as your child begins climbing the stairs, going both up and down.
- Climbing up the stairs precedes descent, and children may find themselves stuck in the middle of the staircase.
- Gradually reduce the support you provide as your child gains proficiency.
- Supervise your child from behind during the climb and from several steps below as your child descends.
- Be ready to catch your child if a misstep or lapse in attention occurs.

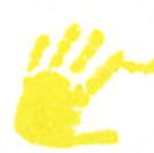

Notes

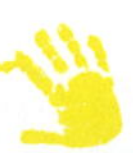

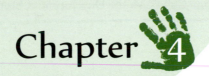

Chapter 4

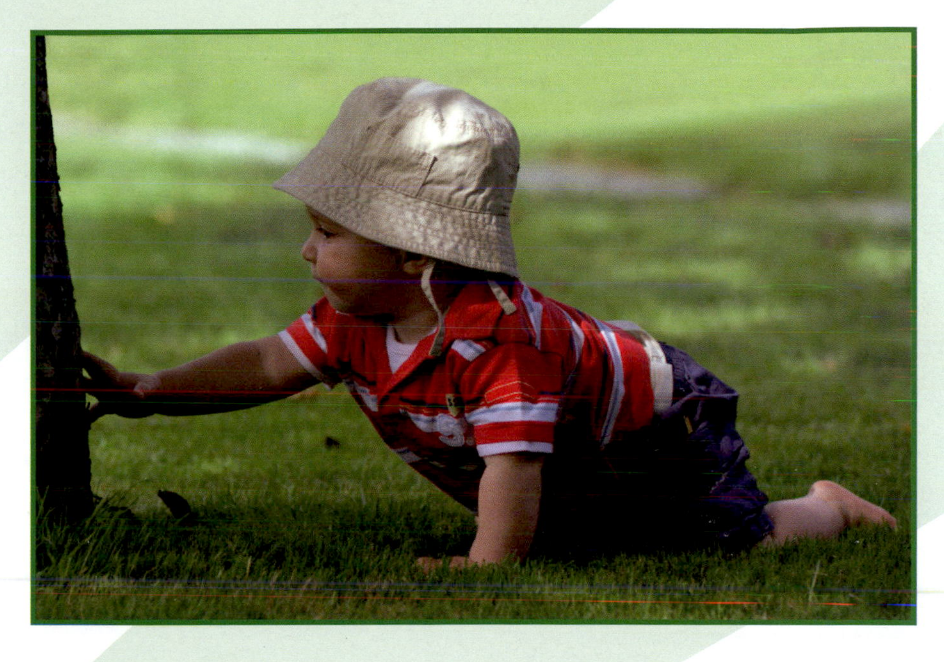

Other Motor Skills Develop— Infancy through Preschool

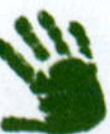

When Jordan was in the first grade, he was referred to me because he had not yet established a preferred hand. His teacher reported seeing him write with his left hand, use scissors with his right, and use either hand to draw, frequently switching back and forth. His parents said that utensil use was random, as well, and that Jordan ate with either hand.

When I sat down with Jordan, I saw that when a crayon was placed on the left side of the desk, he would reach for it with his left hand. When it was placed on the right side, he grasped it with his right hand. Then I had Jordan stand at the chalkboard. He was instructed to stand in one place and draw a horizontal line as far as he could reach. He picked up the chalk and began to draw a line. When Jordan reached the middle, he transferred the chalk to his other hand to complete the line. I then asked him to complete a puzzle on the floor. He was instructed to sit with his legs crossed and reach to the sides to obtain the puzzle pieces. Jordan immediately shifted his position so that the pieces were in front of him. When I attempted to correct him, he again squirmed around to avoid reaching across the midline of his body. Jordan's trunk was not strong. It took a great deal of effort for him to reach. As a result, it was easier for him to grasp objects and manipulate them with whichever hand was closest.

Along with trunk-strengthening activities, Jordan began doing many activities throughout the day that required the use of both hands. He was instructed to use both hands to rub himself down with a towel after a bath. He helped his mom in the kitchen by cleaning the table and countertops with a big sponge, using both hands to wipe back and forth like a windshield wiper, thereby forcing him to cross his midline over and over again. After an intensive month of "extreme bilateral engagement," reaching across his body became automatic and more comfortable. Without the added physical fatigue, he was able to recognize which hand felt better when he drew and practiced letters. Jordan's teacher kept track of his preferences, and, eventually, one hand surfaced as the preferred hand.

While walking takes center stage as a baby grows, many other motor skills are also developing. The arms and hands are

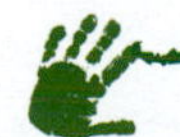

getting stronger. The eyes begin to direct a baby's movements. Both sides of the body begin to work in a coordinated way. The use of the eyes and hands and coordination of movement establish the underpinnings necessary for the development of all skilled movements of the preschooler, student, athlete, and well-functioning adult.

Now let's talk about other motor areas that are developing simultaneously with the skills that lead to walking, as well as ways to enhance the development of these areas. Hand development and fine-motor control emerge over the course of the first year, and a baby's eyes begin to direct the movement of his hands and most motor-based activities. Bilateral skills play an increasingly more important role as the child's movements become more directed and skilled.

As your child's legs have grown stronger over the first 2 years of life, so too have his arms. With walking, his upper extremities play a supporting role. However, most sports require active engagement of his upper body and, in particular, his arms and hands. For that matter, active engagement in almost every task requires the coordinated use of both hands. Anyone who has broken an arm recalls the difficulty in attempting to tie a shoe, button a shirt, open a container, and get toothpaste onto the toothbrush.

Hand and finger dexterity, or *fine-motor skills,* grow alongside gross-motor development. In many ways, they develop in synchrony—improvement in one leads to increased growth in the other. For instance, as your child's hand control increases, he becomes more interested in playing with toys that require reaching. This requires added work from his trunk. As your child stretches to reach for a toy, weight-bearing in his arms and hands occurs, thereby strengthening the muscles in his shoulders, forearms, hands, and fingers. There is a positive synergistic relationship of growth in each area.

Imagine your baby playing with a truck on the floor. While he's sitting, reaching forward or to his side may lead to falling into a four-point or crawling position. Reaching for and pushing the truck while in this position exercises all his trunk muscles and challenges them to react so he can maintain a sense of equilibrium.

When your baby is placed on his tummy, as the truck gets

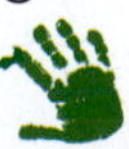

pushed away, a scooting, pulling, or pushing of his whole body occurs to retrieve the vehicle. Once again, heavy work activates his muscles, and all kinds of good information flows into his brain for neurological organization.

As your baby works to obtain the truck, the muscles in his body, arms, and hands get stronger. He learns to move in new ways. His eyes get better at directing movement. Both sides of his body must be engaged to reach the toy successfully.

When I worked in a hospital many years ago, I would enter the elevator in my white lab coat, holding a large exercise ball. This was long before exercises like Pilates had become well known, and these balls had yet to become a fixture in the fitness realm. Looks of puzzlement always greeted me. To begin with, hospitals were not the proper place for playthings, and second, my job was to help patients work on their fine-motor skills. These balls could be found in the physical-therapy gyms but were not recognized as part of an occupational-therapist's

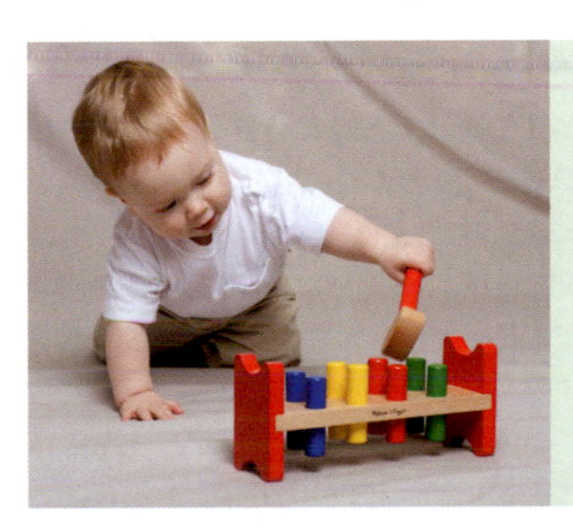

Figure 54. (a) The maturing grasp. **(b)** A "gross grasp," or holding items with the whole fist, is characteristic of very young children.

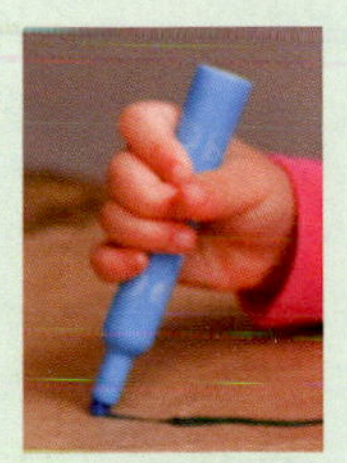

arsenal.

While the rationale is somewhat technical, suffice it to say that therapists had discovered that individuals need to develop solid trunk control to be able to increase fine-motor coordination, whether the difficulty stems from a stroke, a neurological condition, or a weakness from an illness. In addition, strengthening of the arms and hands occurs more effectively through weight-bearing activities.

So, from the halls of the university hospitals to the corridors of many school settings, I towed my exercise balls to treatment sessions. Getting the grown-ups and children alike down on the floor, working against gravity while bearing weight on their hands, became a staple of my treatment sessions.

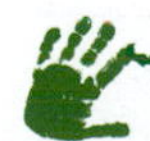

Figure 55. As the fingers get stronger, each finger begins to work on its own with "isolated movement." In this picture, Elisa pushes the Cheerio with her thumb into the side of her index finger. This is called a "lateral pinch."

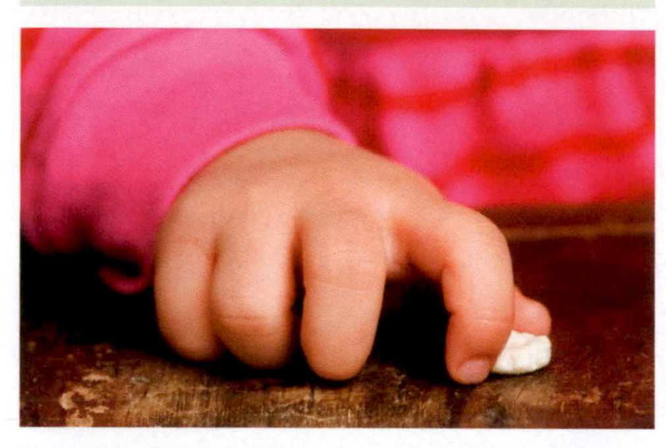

During the first year of a child's life, the development of grasping moves from a fisted hand or "gross" grasp to being able to delicately pick up a small object between the thumb and the tip of the index finger **(Figure 54)**. In between, the baby "palms" objects, which refers to raking objects into the hand with all four fingers. A typical picture of *palming* is when a baby rakes Cheerios into his hand and clasps them with his whole fist.

Grasp becomes more refined when a baby pushes the Cheerios with his thumb against the side of a bent index finger to pick them up. This is called *lateral pinching* **(Figure 55)**.

As your child's thumbs and fingers strengthen, he begins to use his fingertips. Initially, any of the four fingertips may be used. As the thumb gets stronger, it opposes the second and third fingers (index and middle) more consistently. This three-point pinch is called a *three-jaw chuck* grasp. With further strengthening of the thumb and index-finger muscles, your child begins to use his thumb and pointer finger almost exclusively. This is called a *pincer grasp* and is essential for many refined small-motor activities **(Figures 56-58)**.

The variability in grasp development can be seen when

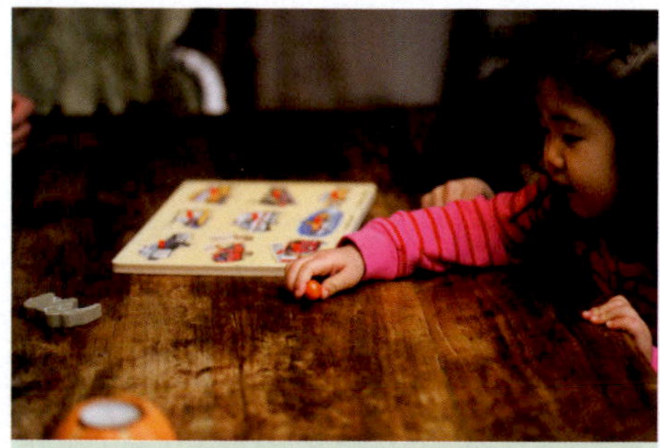

Figure 56. Elisa holds the bead between her thumb and index finger. This reflects a maturing pinch.

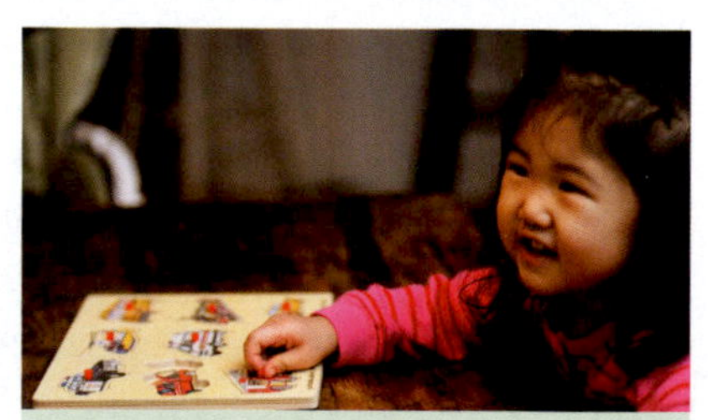

Figure 57. With a good sense of touch, Elisa can feel her fingers touching the knob on the puzzle piece, and she doesn't have to look at her fingers the whole time to be able to guide them.

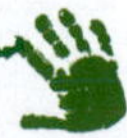

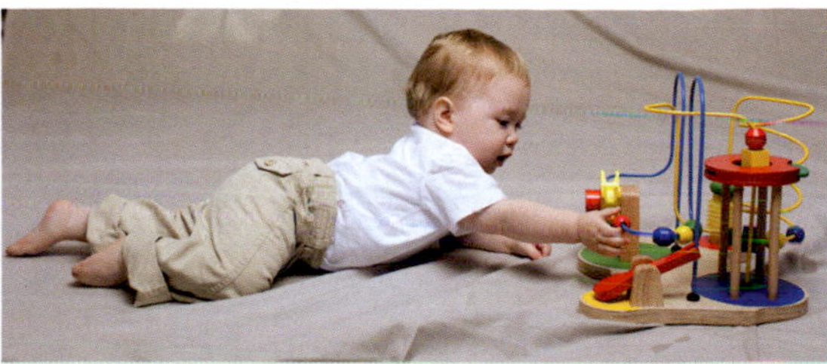

Figure 58. Holding a round bead is more difficult than holding a flat one. It becomes even trickier when the bead moves. Harrison is doing a nice job of holding this round bead while he moves it.

young children are together in a group. Imagine the following scenario at a daycare center. Four 6-month-old babies are sitting in high chairs, waiting for Cheerios to be poured onto their trays. Henry would swipe his arm back and forth over the tray until every Cheerio had fallen to the floor. Tracy would place her chunky little hand on top of the pile and then bend her fingers into her palm. She'd take the fisted booty to her mouth, attempting to smash the Cheerios in, with many falling into her lap. Todd made neat little piles by pushing the cereal toward his fisted hand with his thumb. Olivia gracefully retrieved each piece of cereal between her thumb and fingertip and daintily put it in her mouth, one by one.

Hand development and the refinement of grasp occur at different times for each child—hence the disparity seen between each of these children. Note that each step toward more refined grasping requires "strengthening" of the fingers.

Table 5. Grasping Patterns: A Typical Progression

Step in the Grasping Pattern	Age Seen
Grasp reflex	0-4 months
Intentional gross grasp	3 months
Raking or palming	5 months
Lateral pinch	9 months
Three-jaw chuck grasp	10 months
Pincer grasp	12 months

Note: This Table serves as a general guide. There is great variability in when each child accomplishes these holding patterns.

Tennis pros might use special hand exercisers, but the strengthening of a child's hand should occur naturally. When adequate movement and exploratory opportunities are present, muscles get the exercise they need to become stronger.

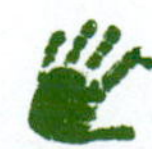

The past three chapters have discussed weight-bearing over and over again. This generally includes bearing weight with the hands (crawling, pushing up from sitting to standing, and playing with toys while lying on the tummy). As a baby's weight is shifted onto his hands, his joints and muscles are stimulated. This stimulation leads to strengthening all of the muscles in his arms, hands, and fingers.

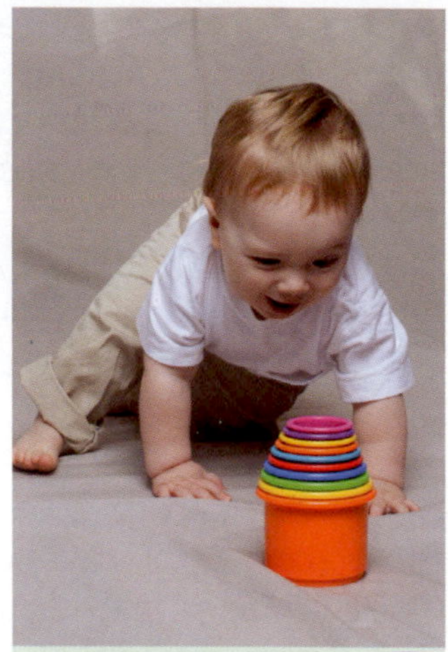

Figure 59. Simple hand strengthening activities. Weight-bearing remains very important for strengthening muscles in the hands and fingers. The longer a baby crawls, the better!

Rory was referred to me at 5 years old because he had trouble holding a pencil. While a child should not be engaged in grueling workbook drills at this age, complete avoidance of coloring and drawing by the time kindergarten starts often indicates some fine- or visual-motor difficulty. When discussing Rory's interests with his mother, she reported that he loved action figures and spent hours playing with characters that required intricate manipulations. Fine-motor control had never been a concern for her.

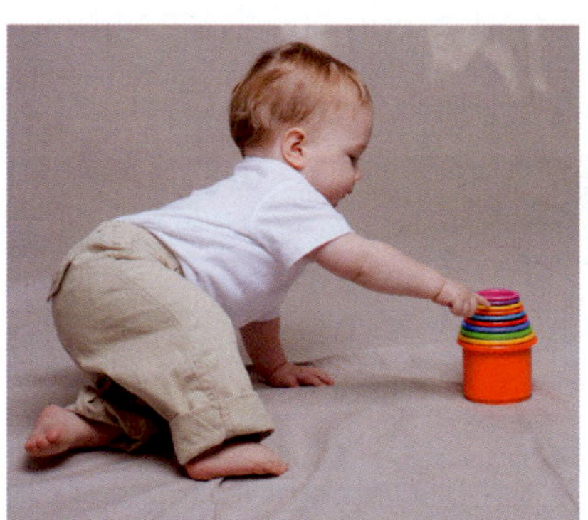

Figure 60. Poking, especially with the index or pointer finger, teaches the finger to move independently of the others. Encourage your child to point at objects and wiggle his pointer finger to increase the movement and strength in this very important finger.

Assessment revealed that Rory had excellent prehension (grasping) patterns. He grasped small objects discretely between his thumb and the tip of his index finger. When he had to exert any force, however, such as pushing to get an object firmly in place, Rory pressed with his thumb against the side of his index finger (a lateral pinch). If that didn't work, he tried to push the object against his chest or the floor.

While these adaptive strategies frequently worked, they reflected a lack of strength in Rory's fingers, which was necessary for

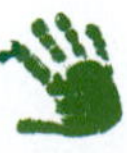

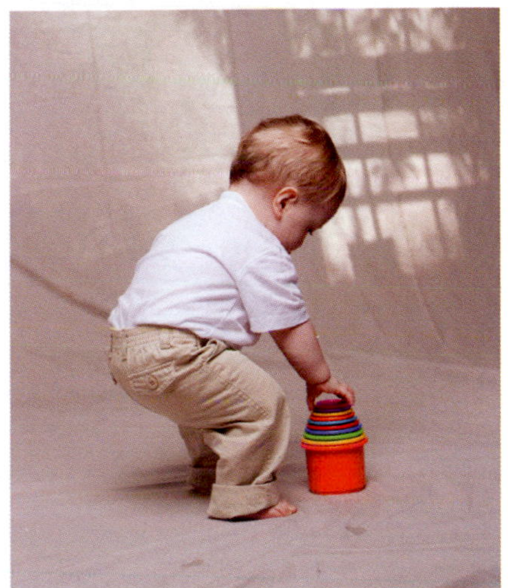

Figure 61. Grasping objects with an outstretched hand begins to strengthen the small muscles in the fingers. These nesting cups require Harrison's hand to stretch varying amounts, because each cup is a different size. Nesting toys like this can be found at stores for less than 10 dollars. However, cleaned peanut butter jars and lids, which facilitate twisting, are even better!

complex manipulations. Drawing requires holding a pencil with the fingertips. The fingers need to be able to move and exert force at the same time. Rory hadn't acquired the strength necessary to execute the push-and-pull types of motions required for drawing and early writing.

Each time a baby's hands open and close, muscles activate and strengthen. Each time an object is grasped, the muscles strengthen. When toys of varying shapes, sizes, and weights are introduced, new groups of muscle fibers get stronger. When a child opens his hand wide to feel a textured object, the extensor muscles are activated. When a child holds a toy with his fingers partially bent, extensor and flexor muscles have to work cooperatively to strengthen both groups. Little muscles deep within the hand also begin to work.

Hand games, such as "Where Is Thumbkin," in which the thumb pops up and wiggles around, or "Open, Shut Them," in which the hands open and close, help strengthen varying muscle groups and teach the fingers to move independently **(Figures 59-62)**.

Developing fine-motor skills does not require a sophisticated cache of toys or lessons. A child should play with safe, familiar objects around the house. Allow playtime with pots and pans, measuring cups and spoons, plastic containers, clean jars with screw-on caps, and a variety of other items. These enable the child to explore, feel, and grasp objects in ways that develop and strengthen the hands.

Common issues with hand-strengthening relate to how well the thumb can move away from the hand and if the tip of the

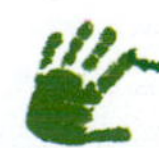

thumb can bend and exert force when strength is required. Since babies start out with tightly fisted hands, the natural and most comfortable position for the thumb is tucked into the side of the hand. The muscles pulling the thumb in (adductor muscles) are strongest. It is the job of the child to strengthen the muscles that pull the thumb away from the palm (abductor muscles). Great activities to help strengthen the abductor muscles are using spray bottles and working with scissors. Children I work with frequently are assigned spray-bottle work (such as spraying plants) for 5 minutes every day. Their thumb needs to stretch around the bottle top, while their fingers stretch over the nozzle that is being squeezed. When the tip of their thumb is hyperextended or bends backward, I encourage the child to go back to using simple squeezing and grasping toys until their hands get stronger. Hand-play activities that require the tip of the thumb to be used are helpful.

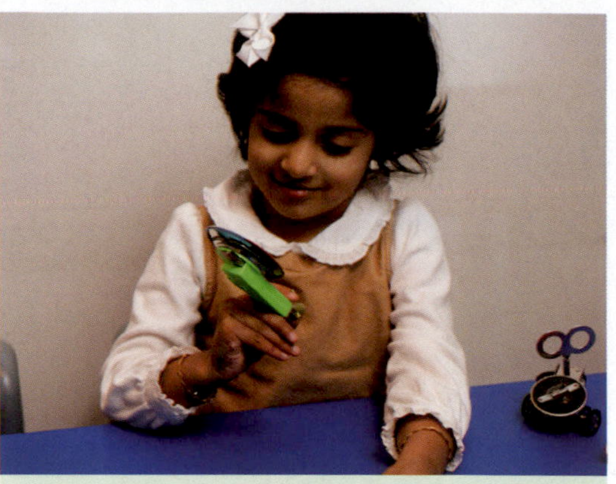

Figure 62. By 4 years old, the hand should be getting stronger, and the child can begin concentrating on more sophisticated activities, such as playing with wind-up toys and objects that require some manipulation. The sparkler toy pictured here requires the thumb to push a lever back and forth to make the wheel move. The rotating wheel drags over a rough surface. This causes friction, which creates sparks, or "sparkles." Along with a lesson in physics, this simple toy strengthens the muscles in the thumbs and teaches the fingers to do individual jobs (the thumb moves while the fingers hold the toy steady).

Spray bottles, squeeze bottles, and supervised button-pushing (eg, coffee grinders, blenders) all require special work with the hands. Deep muscles in the fingers are activated, which strengthen the muscles required for sophisticated movements in the hands and fingers. Squeezing sponges and crumpling and ripping paper all provide wonderful hand manipulation opportunities, as well.

Pointing an index finger and poking with it help to strengthen it. Using shaving cream or foamy soap in the bathtub and

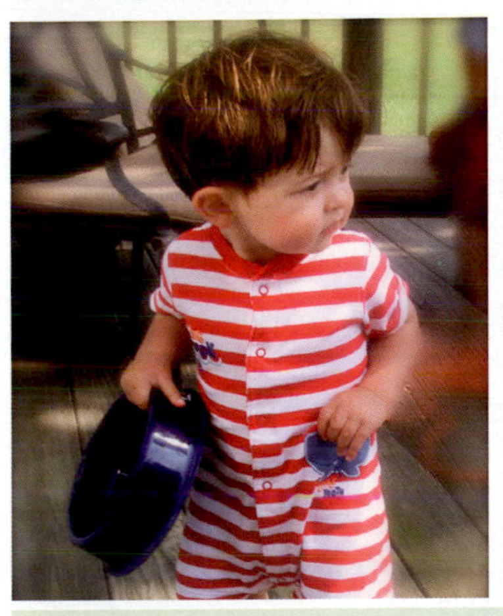

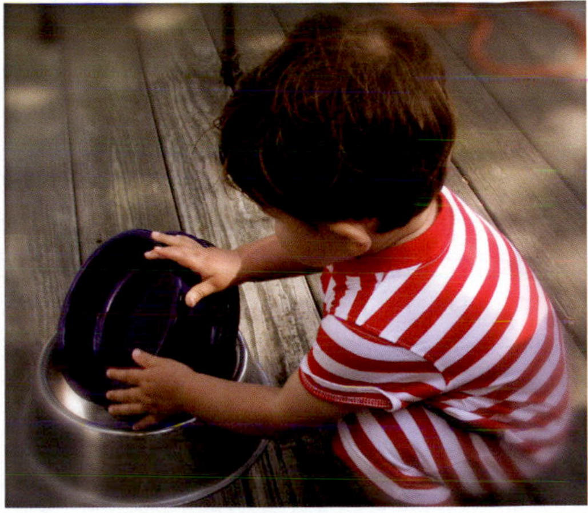

Figure 63. (a) Visiting from California, Pedrito doesn't need an arsenal of toys to play with. He takes delight in stacking dog bowls while his mom and dad chat with friends. **(b)** While he is in his own little world playing with these newfound delights, adults are close by to make sure he only plays with things that are safe.

making scribble pictures with the whole hand and pointed index finger are examples of ways to strengthen the fingers and hands. Or, you could do the same with pudding on a highchair tray.

Picking up little objects (large enough to be safe and not swallowed if put in the mouth) of varying sizes and shapes helps refine the three-jaw chuck grasp and pincer grasp. Spoons, keys, and erasers are just a few examples. Manipulating food provides wonderful opportunities for developing grasping proficiency. Cheerios are universally employed. Cut 1-inch cubes rather than slices of cheese and meat once the child can manage chewing and swallowing them to facilitate a fingertip grasp. Do the same with fruits and vegetables.

At one point, I had 12-month-old twins and a very active 4-year-old. Imagine the potential struggle of cooking dinner without help! Fortunately, I had a corner cabinet that housed all my pots and pans. It also entertained my three children for the duration of the nightly preparations. First they dragged each item out of the cabinet, banging it, stacking it, nesting it, and exploring the features of each one. Then they took turns crawling into the empty cabinet space. While I might not have created a gourmet "Julia Child" dinner, I had the time to throw a meal together with minimal interruptions.

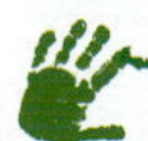

While I cooked, my children organically learned valuable lessons in size and weight variability (lifting, nesting, and stacking pots), developed bilateral motor coordination (crashing lids together like cymbals), and increased the strength of their fingers (grasping all these objects). Finger dexterity improved as they poked their little fingers into various holes and ridges. Coordination increased as they attempted to put things together and take them apart. They also had the opportunity to develop their imaginations as they crawled into the seemingly cavernous cabinet space.

After preparing dinner, I was left with a huge mess of pots and pans scattered about the room. It took about 5 minutes to reassemble them and put them back in the cabinet, which I was more than happy to do.

As fine-grasping patterns emerge and develop, a child becomes aware of how to move and use her arms, hands, and fingers. This segues into manipulating objects successfully. Proficiency leads to greater enjoyment when playing with toys. This extends the child's attention span and begins to build a firm understanding of cause and effect.

Successful play leads to a sense of competence and autonomy. The ability to manage the objects in one's environment gives an individual a sense of control and an understanding of how the physical world works. This, in general, is critical to developing an overall ability to perform in the world **(Figure 63)**.

Recommended Activities

- Provide opportunities for your baby to touch objects and varied surfaces soon after birth. Offering a finger for her to squeeze and gently opening her hand to rub soft surfaces begins a lifelong exploratory process.
- As her hand begins to open voluntarily, provide interesting shapes of different sizes and textures to hold with assistance.
- Play simple hand games, such as "Open, Shut Them," "How Big Is...," and "Bye-Bye," in which her little hands learn to move in specific ways.
- When her fingers begin to move independently, encourage pointing and poking with her index finger.

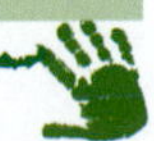

- Play thumb games, such as "Where Is Thumbkin?"
- As her hands and fingers get stronger, provide opportunities to poke and press with her thumb and index finger in a functional way. Examples include pressing buttons on small kitchen appliances, such as a blender or mixer, with supervision.
- When holding hands, play the "Squeeze Game." You and your child take turns increasing the pressure and squeezing each other's hand.
- Manipulative toys should be large enough so your child's fingers have to stretch across the surface slightly, thereby working the flexor and extensor muscles of the fingers at the same time. Duplos and wooden alphabet blocks are perfectly sized toys for a toddler's hands.
- Perfect activities to do prior to using scissors and drawing tools include employing a spray bottle or a large sponge. Your child can play in the tub with these items or even help you by "cleaning" tabletops with water and watering plants.
- Weight-bearing activities, such as wheelbarrow-walking and crab-walking, help build strength in the arms and small muscles of your child's hands.
- Once your child is old enough to use tools, activities that involve the use of scissors and wooden stamps will strengthen the muscles necessary for drawing and writing. Picking up playing cards with the fingertips and manipulating the cards when dealing them or fanning them out also activate muscles in a maturing preschooler's hands.

In the Eyes of the Beholder

No matter what the activity—whether playing outside or with a sports team, pursuing artistic endeavors, or simply taking care of personal business such as dressing and eating—the hands and eyes work as a team to accomplish each task. Of course, there are remarkable exceptions to this rule. A visually challenged individual copes with blindness by refining his other senses to compensate. Normally, however, vision plays a key role in guiding the hands and body to do the work needed to accomplish most tasks successfully.

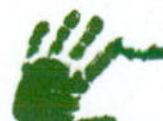

Using the eyes to guide motor-based activities seems apparent and obvious. The assumption that vision automatically accompanies movement in children is erroneous, however. Shoe sales attendants recount stories of children attempting to shove their feet into shoes without looking for several minutes before the clerk intervenes. Teachers observe many children painting blissfully, eyes wandering all over the room while gobs of paint drip off the brush and easel. Likewise, the accident-prone child, tripping around the playground, is often simply "not looking where he is going." There are many components that lead to the automatic linking of visually directed motor activity.

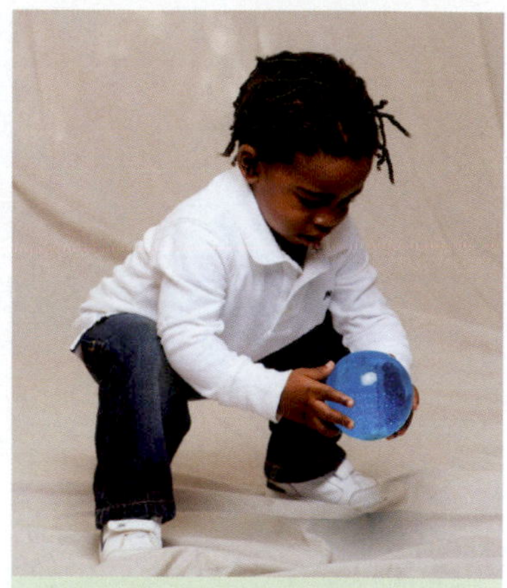

Figure 64. Developing visual focus at an early age leads to the visual skills necessary to play many sports, read, write, and pay attention to what's going on in our environment. In essence, our visual focus assists us with everything we do throughout the day!

Remember when you held your newborn baby in your arms? Every once in a while, your child's eyes met yours, and you gazed lovingly at one another. Gradually, your prolonged eye contact became more frequent. Your baby began to associate you and your face with the positive feelings that came from being held securely, hearing your soft voice, and experiencing your comforting touch. Over time, your baby learned to follow your voice and your movement around the room.

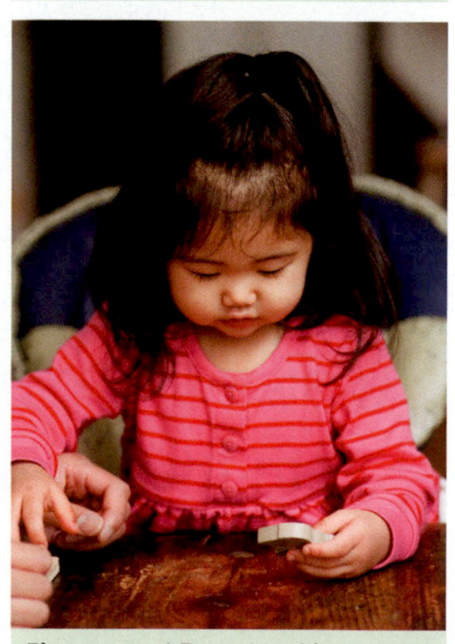

Figure 65. Looking at interesting objects up close, such as looking at picture books, helps facilitate visual attention. When holding an interesting toy, a child begins to integrate the hand-eye connection.

Now think of the way a young baby plays. When a rattle is jiggled on a baby's left or right side, her head and arm will move simultaneously in the direction of the noise. As a very young infant, the movement of her arm automatically moves her

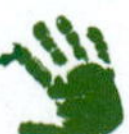

head, while her eyes look out toward her hand (called the *fencing reflex,* which we discussed in chapter 1).

As your infant gazes into your face, her *visual focus* begins to develop. When your baby's eyes follow the movements of others around the room, nascent *visual tracking* begins. While she's playing, and her arm moves with her head and eyes following it, a rudimentary *eye-hand connection* is made. When you snap your fingers on her right side and then quickly switch to her left, causing her to look back and forth, rapid eye shifts called *saccadic eye movements* also develop.

At first, your newborn's eye and head movements seem random. Over time, her eyes and head begin to move intentionally toward sounds and visual images.

Refinement of that intentional eye movement improves over time in several ways:

Gaze: The eyes look intently at one point of interest.

Tracking: The eyes follow a moving target.

Focusing: The eyes gaze at a single point.

Saccadic movement: The eyes shift from one point to another rapidly.

Binocularity: The two eyes are used in a coordinated way **(Figures 64 and 65)**.

How Does Vision Relate to "The Motor Story?"

To begin with, our eyes are capable of movement because we have muscles attached to our eyeballs, allowing us to move them around. Our arms bend and straighten because our biceps and triceps muscles move the bones in our forearms. Similarly, our vision is dependent on the muscular activity of our eyes for independent movement. Extraocular muscles, or the muscles attached to our eyeballs, help our eyes to move and move together in a coordinated way.

Depth perception depends upon the coordinated move-

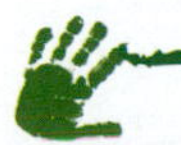

ment of both eyes, or *binocular vision*. When the vision in one eye is impaired, it is more difficult to determine the distances of objects. For example, going down an unfamiliar staircase might be scary if your depth perception were affected. Determining the distance your foot needs to move to reach the next step becomes difficult without adequate depth perception.

The muscles around the eyes develop to be able to move them in a coordinated way. Muscle strength and coordination are key components in visual tracking, binocularity, and focusing. The eye muscles need to develop, just as the small muscles of the hands and fingers must develop to push a pencil around successfully.

While engaged in motor tasks, we learn to shift the gaze of our eyes. Remember when Ashley ran across the parking lot and could not respond to her mother's call? Walking took up all of Ashley's focus and energy. Moving her eyes and head to look at a new target was beyond her motor capacity at that time. All her energy was focused on the task of walking, and she could not shift her gaze from a single visual target. For her, safety in the parking lot did not come into her awareness, because she needed to focus exclusively on walking.

How Does the Integration of Movement and the Ability to Visually Attend Occur?

Let's begin with a fairly sedentary activity, such as looking at a picture book. A young child usually sits in one position while her eyes look at one small area (the book). The only demand on her body is to maintain an upright position. For your baby, even this ability is reduced when being held in your lap. Your baby's visual field is limited to the pages of the book. The only other motor demand may be turning the pages.

Think of the popularity of certain children's books. Richard Scarry became fabulously successful as he recognized the intrigue and delightful challenge of looking at a large page filled with familiar images of everyday life. A child could focus on the small details of a truck and move her eyes a few inches

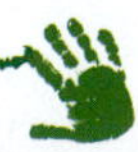

to see a train chugging along. Further along the page, the familiar and comforting image of the mommy bear holding her baby cub comes into view.

The task of reading is even more complicated. This requires the child to look at very small targets (letters) and then move her eyes in a specific direction. Reading is generally not considered a motor activity. Yet, the small-motor demands required to read successfully are quite significant. The eyes must focus acutely on one spot and then move small distances to see each letter. This requires the eyes to stay steady, move horizontally across a page (tracking), then shift downward slightly and quickly back to the opposite side (saccadic movement) to begin the sequence again.

As your child learns to read, it is a stop-and-start, halting process as words are sounded out. Pointing with a finger or using a marker often helps your child focus in the early stages of reading. As she progresses in her reading ability and the capacity of her eyes to look at words improves, the flow of tracking and the amount of visual information packaged in each glance improves, as well.

Writing is a demanding visual task. Like reading, the eyes must follow the letters written. However, a second motor task (moving the pencil) must be coordinated simultaneously. One hand moves the pencil, while the other hand holds the paper still. While this bilateral task is occurring, the eyes must direct the writing hand in the path it must take (eg, drawing a circle for an "O") and verify that the letter is written correctly.

Stephanie was referred to me at 5 years old. She was a bright little girl who had already begun to read. The referral form indicated that Stephanie struggled with a pencil. She held the pencil correctly, but when she was asked to copy simple shapes, Stephanie looked around the classroom as she scribbled random lines on the page. She hadn't made the connection that her eyes were supposed to tell her hands where to go. We spent time playing catch and batting at balloons until she understood that her eyes needed to follow her hands to be successful. We also played several fine-motor games that required her eyes to direct the movement. Over time, Stephanie "got it," and her eyes automatically followed her hands as she drew and learned to copy letters.

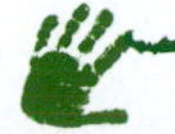

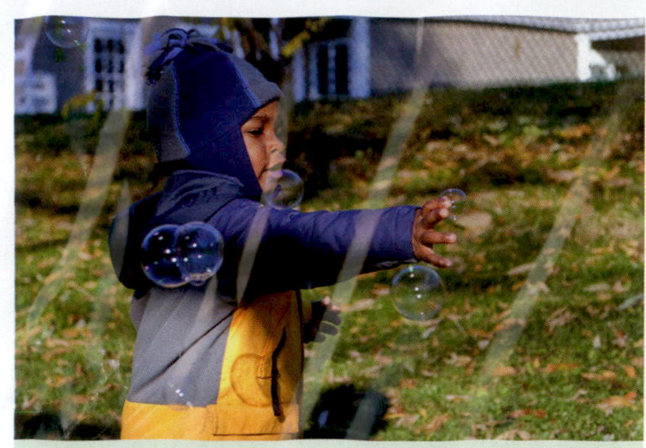

Figure 66. Wayne catches bubbles while standing still, demonstrating dynamic visual tracking. Bubbles move slowly, so they are easy to follow and catch.

Reading requires a coordination of eye movements and the ability of the body to stay in a fairly stable position. Writing adds hand movements to the visual-motor task, so the coordination of eye and body movements increases.

Now let's move onto the playground and consider the many visual-motor demands required of a toddler and preschooler to run around and negotiate the equipment successfully!

First, your toddler must be able to observe objects in the play yard. His visual field has expanded from *near-point* or *central/focal vision* to *peripheral vision*. Identifying structures to be able to move around them and determining how far away they are is a first step. More complex is determining how to cope with moving objects, such as other children. Your child may set out for the swing set, but along the way, another child darts out into the intended pathway. At this moment, your toddler must alter course by either stopping or moving around the other child. If this decision is not made, a collision is likely to occur.

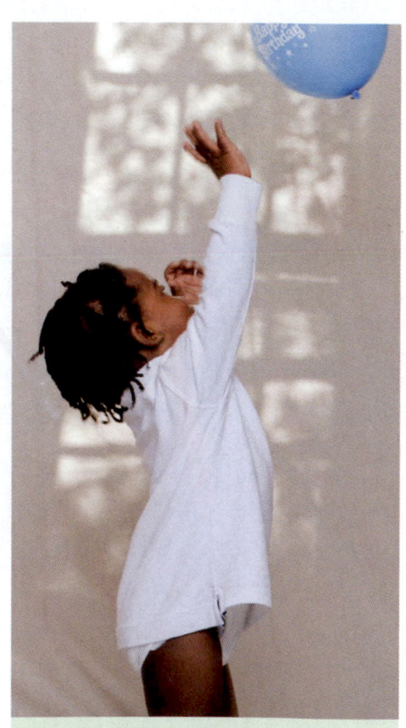

Figure 67. Wayne runs up to a balloon and reaches out to bat at it. Balloons are another kind of slow-moving object that makes it easy for a child to look at it, move toward it, and touch it.

Interaction with moving objects is yet another demand. As mentioned previously, determining how to move around a child that is interfering with an intended pathway begins the more dynamic aspect of "work" on

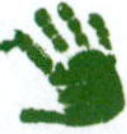

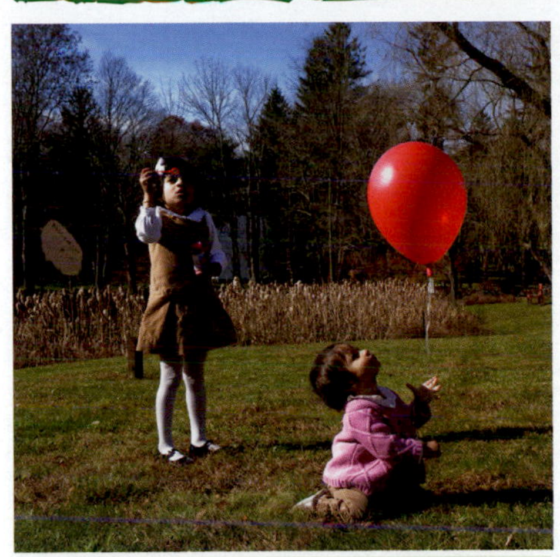

Figure 68. Compare the sophistication of the 4-year-old's visual attention to that of a 10-month-old. Aanya (4 years) is able to hold the bottle, blow bubbles, and watch them as they float away. Vedha (10 months) looks with intent at the big red balloon. She works at holding the string (fortunately it is tied to her wrist). Big bright objects hold the attention of a younger child. As the child grows, intricate details and the more dynamic nature of visual stimuli begin to hold the child's attention.

the playground. Figuring out how run away from other children is another. This requires an integration of keeping visual focus on the new friend and moving in a specified way.

Playing with a ball is another visually demanding activity. This process should begin slowly and long before your baby can walk. The simple back-and-forth play of rolling a truck or ball sets the stage for developing ball-handling skills later on.

As your baby lies or sits on the floor, you can slowly roll a ball to him. He will grasp the ball as it arrives or even push it back. This back-and-forth activity facilitates eye-hand coordination. He readies his arms for the oncoming ball as his eyes follow its movement. Finally, he observes his hand making contact with the ball. His eyes assist in directing his arm to push the ball away or grasp the ball for further exploration.

Balloons and bubbles offer similar experiences **(Figures 66 and 67)**. They move slowly through the air, allowing a child to follow the movement as it approaches. If the child bats at it successfully, the balloon or bubble lurches away, thereby extending the visual activity.

These simple activities usually produce gleeful reactions from children. The bright colors and slower pacing of these objects are easier to see and track, allowing a child to feel successful in the early acquisition of eye-hand skills.

Bubbles and balloons segue into softballs, baseballs, footballs, tennis balls, soccer balls, and more. The size, color, and speed of these different kinds of "toys" demand greater at-

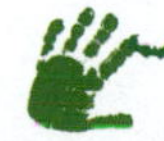

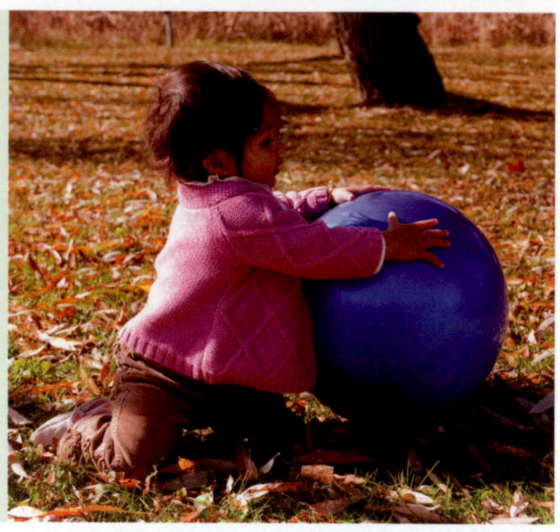

Figure 69. For activities to encourage crossing the midline, inexpensive, brightly colored balls are a favorite. Because of the size of the ball, Vedha is reaching across the midline of her body in an attempt to grasp the ball with both hands.

tention, focusing, and agility of the eyes to be able to follow the target **(Figures 68 and 69)**. Intermediate toys such as foam, Gertie balls, and beanbags provide a bridge to more sophisticated eye-hand demands. These allow your child to practice the developing skill of tracking an object like a ball, right to the point when it reaches her hands as it's caught.

Now think of a child standing in the outfield, arms open wide and at the ready, gloved hand extended, shouting, "I've got it, I've got it!" until the ball falls with a thud 10 feet away. This Little Leaguer hasn't integrated the ability to watch, anticipate, move, and then catch the ball.

In this scenario, moving to the ball requires several elements. First, the child must watch the visual target (the ball) as it moves. Second, the child must move toward the ball. The hands must simultaneously prepare to catch the speeding orb as it falls toward the earth. This is a complex skill that continues to develop as the child grows. Some adults would argue that they continue working on this throughout life! Ask any recreational tennis player about the importance of "keeping an eye on the ball."

Our visual attention continues to direct all our movements. Ski instructors suggest that skiers look 10 to 20 feet ahead and never at the skis or the terrain immediately before them. With this visual guidepost, a skier's movements become automatic and smooth and acquire a rhythm. Yoga and Pilates instructors remind their students to find one visual focal point when

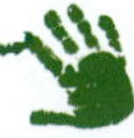

balancing. The challenge occurs when they are asked to then shift their gaze. Suddenly, the static position the student is holding teeters until focus is regained and a sense of center is reestablished.

Maintaining visual focus while the body moves affects many activities. Consider golf. When you swing a golf club, your eyes must remain on the little white ball as your body twists and your arms swing to launch the ball off the tee. If your eyes leave the ball (to see how well it's been hit), your stroke immediately shifts, and a perfect shot is ruined. When a tennis player plans a perfect put-away volley but looks at the intended target rather than at the ball, an error usually occurs. In basketball, a player must focus on a target, such as the rim, to make the shot. Even while the ball is being dribbled, lifted, and shot toward the hoop, the player's eyes never leave the target. These examples illustrate the discipline required to stay visually focused.

Each sport also requires an acute awareness of how the body is positioned and moving. Being able to precisely move certain body parts and keep others perfectly still while visually focusing reflects the culmination of the development of visual-motor integration, bilateral coordination, and eye-hand coordination.

These examples indicate that the effective use of vision requires a coordination of motor and visual skills on many levels. The ability to sit at a desk and use your eyes effectively for reading and word-processing is one aspect of vision. The ability to stand and watch a moving target requires another level of visual-motor integration. Learning to run and catch a ball requires even further sophistication of vision and motor coordination. Being able to execute a movement with your focus glued to a specific target while the rest of your body moves, as is required to hit a golf ball correctly, demands an even higher level of discipline and coordination of motor and visual control.

Meeting the increasing complexity and demands of visual-motor coordination occurs through the establishment of the many building blocks already discussed. Strong core strength throughout the trunk provides a stable base. The body can then develop isolated movements, such as moving the arms while the head stays trained in one direction. Strong head and neck control, which we discussed earlier, facilitates good mus-

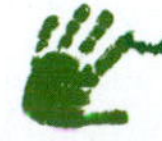

cle control of the eyes. Additionally, varied movement experiences lead to improved depth perception.

As your child develops nice grasping patterns and learns to use his hands in a coordinated way, habituated movements develop. Your child no longer has to focus on how to move his fingers to complete a task. This frees up his eyes so he no longer has to look at and direct every movement of the hands. Instead, his eyes can focus on the bigger picture. As proficiency in gross- and fine-motor skills increases, more attention can be directed toward the surrounding environment—whether on the playing field or in the classroom.

My work as a clinician spans several decades. As a result, I have had the pleasure of working with children at various stages in their motor development. I worked with Mary when she struggled with writing as a first grader. She learned to carefully direct the pencil with her eyes for each downward and circular stroke. Her success in writing the letter "A" depended on this guidance. During therapy, repetition in drawing the strokes necessary for each letter eventually led to ease in copying the alphabet. After many years, I had the good fortune to see Mary again as a high-school student preparing to take the SAT writing test. She no longer needed to look at her hands and pencil when she wrote. Her eyes were able to focus on the text written on the chalkboard. Her pencil glided effortlessly across the page as she copied the material from the board. She comfortably scribbled lecture notes she could refer to at a later time.

I also worked with Hunter as a preschooler. He spent a good deal of time learning how to tie his shoes and zip his coat. A major accomplishment was learning to button. He spent 10 minutes every morning buttoning his sweater for school. It was an exercise in determination and pride that he could carefully examine the button held between his fingers, push it through the buttonhole, and have the other hand pull it through. Fast forward to high school. Hunter's mother reports that he buttons his shirt as he runs out the door to catch the bus, looking around to see whether he's made it in time.

From all these building blocks, a child develops the ability to sit and pay attention to the teacher's lesson. A student can look back and forth from the blackboard to his notebook, copiously copying notes. A Little Leaguer learns to catch the ball in the

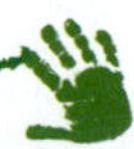

outfield and throw it with accuracy. A football player can scan the field to locate a charging defender, as well as hone in on an oncoming pass. The athlete simultaneously readies his body to move toward the football while preparing his trunk for a major hit.

It may seem a long way from rolling a little red ball into the hands of a toddler to the football coach's unrelenting drill demands, but the objectives are all the same:

1. Strengthen the body, especially the core musculature.
2. Increase flexibility.
3. Develop eye-hand coordination
4. Anticipate through visual assessment.
5. Execute with visual guidance.

Recommended Activities

- The development of visual ability in your newborn begins the moment the two of you share your first gaze.
- Face-to-face contact should continue frequently throughout your baby's waking hours.
- During your baby's alert periods, moving objects in front of him, side to side and up and down, facilitates visual tracking.
- Place objects within striking range to encourage your child to bat things with his hands.
- Situate your child in varied positions, such as on his tummy or in a supported sitting position. Then position toys slightly off center from your baby's visual field so his eyes must move to locate the object. Introduce toys, such as rolling trucks and balls in front of him. These toys require him to follow a moving target.
- As independent movement develops, incorporate push-and-pull toys, such as cars and objects on strings, so your child's hands and eyes sync up with the motor demands of retrieving and moving objects.

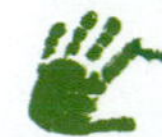

- Reciprocal ball play should begin with objects in slow motion, such as rolled balls and balloons. An inverse relationship of size and speed should occur as his ability improves. For an older child, changing it up with alternate activities, such as throwing Frisbees, provides an additional opportunity to work on visual tracking with a slower moving object.
- Rolling trucks, cars, and trains while crawling should continue for many years. As a preschooler progresses, drawing chalk lines on the ground for roadways not only continues to develop gross-, fine-, and visual-motor development, it also introduces spatial concepts of parallel lines and directionality.
- Opportunities to look at picture books and play with toys, such as stuffed animals, should be interwoven into the fabric of every day. Reading books and playing with toys requires visual focusing more specific than that required when scanning the environment in a general way.
- When talking to a growing child, always give the courtesy of establishing eye contact throughout the conversation. (Note: However, this is difficult and unsafe to do in a car!)
- Games of "I Spy" can be part of many dialogues throughout the day, without the formality of playing an official game. Seeing things that sit still and then suddenly move, such as butterflies and other animals, brings particular joy, in part because they offer the opportunity to visually focus and then track.
- Specific games to augment visual tracking include flashlight tag, simple puppet play, bubbles, ball mazes, and tracking towers.

Note: Video and computer screens are quite small, relative to the visual scope of the real world. Therefore, the development of a child's visual skills related to tracking and saccadic movement in these mediums is quite limited. Remember that when your child is watching a movie, she is also stationary, so the interdependence of body movements and visual integration will not occur.

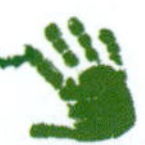

Two Hands Are Better Than One

In my work, children must take their shoes off before playing on the mats. This means they need to put them back on at the end of the session. Dozens of times a day, I observe children twisting and pounding their feet while contorting their bodies in all kinds of interesting ways in an attempt to get their foot into a shoe without using both hands. In broken-record fashion, I relay that they need to use two hands. "It takes team work: two hands, a foot, and two eyes!" Eventually they listen, or I assist with this process. Some activities simply require two hands. The task *may* be executed one handed, but it becomes a labored, inefficient exercise in frustration.

As humans evolved into bipeds (in essence, using two rather than four legs to walk), our arms were freed up to engage in activities in a more sophisticated way. The use of tools developed, and with it, the ability to assign each hand a specific task to make the job easier. The cave man learned that the spear came out of the kill more easily when one hand held the carcass down as the other hand pulled the stick out.

We think of bilateral skill development when talking about playing volleyball and cutting with scissors. Some recognize the bilateral nature of riding a bike or swimming. The arms and legs on both sides of the body have specific jobs to do. Sometimes, the arms do exactly the same thing at the same time, such as when batting a ball, using a rolling pin to roll out dough, or jumping rope. Other times, the right and left do the same thing but in opposite directions, as in running or skipping.

Many activities, such as cutting with scissors, require each hand to do a specific task. Each job compliments the other. In the example of cutting, while one hand moves the scissors, the other hand holds and moves the article intended to be cut.

As discussed earlier, when writing, the preferred hand holds and moves the pencil. The job of the nondominant hand is to hold the paper still. With time, the writer unconsciously anticipates the subtle push and pull of the paper so that equal and opposite force is applied as the pencil moves across the page, thereby preventing any shifting of the paper.

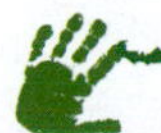

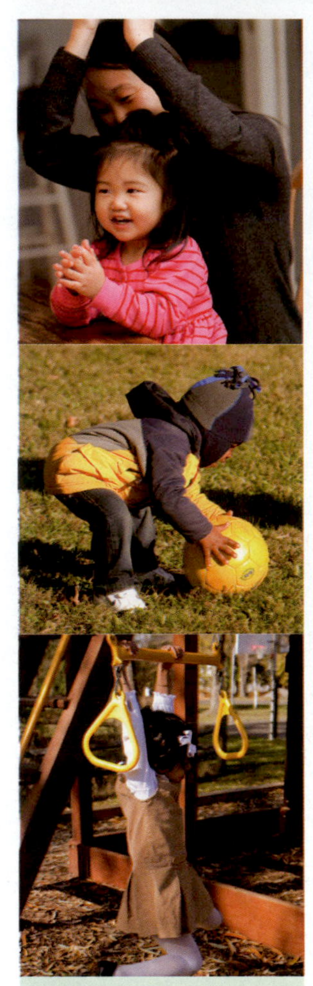

Figure 70. Terrific everyday activities that develop bilateral skills. **(a)** Clapping! **(b)** Ball play is always a favorite. **(c)** Holding on with two hands!

Many of the children I work with hold their heads rather than the paper while they write. As they work, the paper shifts all over the table, leading to a sloppy end product. It also slows down the writing process. Occasionally, I will pull the paper out from under them so they learn the importance of holding down or stabilizing the paper.

Development of bilateral skills originates with the random play of the legs and arms. It becomes refined as the two hands come together for "Pat-a-Cake" and other games **(Figure 70)**. As the legs begin to move in unison and then in a reciprocal way, such as in crawling and walking, bilateral reciprocal patterns are established.

This continues as your child toddles and enters preschool. Many everyday tasks encourage your child to develop bilateral skills. Washing and drying her hands by rubbing both hands together help reinforce the use of both hands. Holding onto a large sponge with two hands to wipe down a table is a simple activity that makes both hands work together. Reciprocal movements occur when the right and left hands beat a drum independently, such as in a rhythmic sequence. Holding a bowl with one hand while the dominant hand stirs is another example. Batting at a balloon with two hands and using a "bopper," such as a cardboard paper towel tube, are fun precursors to using a baseball bat, hockey stick, or racquet.

Catching a ball or Frisbee with two hands precedes a one-handed catch. Two-handed catching requires both hands to come to the midline of the body, a critical aspect of bilateral control. To advance to higher-level athletic skills, a child needs

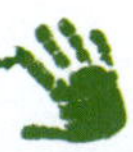

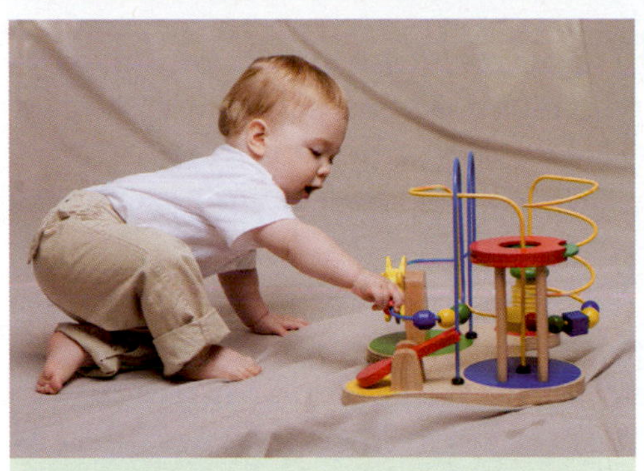

Figure 71. Placing enticing toys to the side of the child while he sits, rather than in front him, encourages him to cross the midline. In his eagerness to play with this toy, Harrison moves from sitting to a transitional position between sitting and crawling.

to be proficient with working at and crossing the midline of the body **(Figure 71)**.

Imagine the picture of a person facing forward, with their arms and legs held slightly out to the sides. Then draw a line from the top of the head straight down through the entire length of the trunk. This constitutes the midline of the body. Exactly half of the body is on the right, including the right arm and leg. The other half, of course, is the entire left side of the body.

Think of the way a baby shakes a favorite stuffed toy. Sometimes the left hand is used, and sometimes the right. Eventually, both hands meet in the middle. Both hands grasp the toy to shake it vigorously. This delights the baby. If the toy inadvertently gets dropped, rapid retrieval allows the child to "practice" reaching with both hands. Happily, with an immediate response, learning to hold a toy with two hands is reinforced.

By positioning a toy directly in front of or at the midline, the baby can choose to grab it with one or both hands. When both the right and left hands grasp, the toy remains directly in the baby's visual field. The enjoyable sensation of shaking the toy is compounded by the ability to see it, as well. A huge leap in bilateral and visual motor development occurs!

Work at the midline of the body begins when the baby's hands touched intentionally. Holding and manipulating toys at the center of the body begin the process of bilateral skill development. Initially, both hands learn to do the same job, such as holding a toy, as described earlier. Later, one hand holds the toy, while the other hand manipulates it.

The next challenge is when objects are placed to the sides of the child rather than in front of her. Reaching across her body, or crossing the midline, such as using her right hand to reach to her left side to retrieve a block, is important for build-

ing the strength and flexibility required for moving the trunk in many directions. Remember Jordan, discussed at the beginning of this chapter? He needed to strengthen his trunk and be able to reach across his body before he could develop a hand preference.

Bilateral skills frequently require a combination of two hands and legs working together. Some activities require the hands and legs to do the same thing at the same time, working in unison. Other times, the limbs engage in a coordinated sequence of reciprocal movements. Sometimes the movements constitute a repetitive movement, as in running or rowing. Other times, it requires a sophisticated understanding of what the dominant side is doing, so the opposite hand can anticipate and make the necessary counterbalancing movement to execute an action successfully. This is employed when hammering a nail—one hand holds the nail and adjusts it accordingly, while the other hand pounds away at it with the hammer. The same mechanism is at work when stabilizing a basketball to make a shot from the foul line.

Recommended Activities

- Bring your newborn's hands and feet together when playing and cuddling with her. The movement and sensation of her two sides touching will heighten her overall awareness of both sides of her body.
- Hand play and simple rhythm games should be incorporated into regular play routines, from babyhood through early grade school. Complexity ranges from clapping and shaking hands and stomping feet to sophisticated jump-rope play and reciprocal hand-clapping sequences with a partner.
- Provide opportunities for reaching across the midline of the body early in development. Have your child reach across her body while she's in a supported sitting position, followed by reaching while independently sitting, crawling, and standing.
- Make sure both her hands are engaged when she's executing most fine- and gross-motor activities. When introducing early gross-motor skills, gently guide and encourage your child to use both hands. For example, have her roll a ball

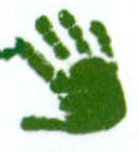

with both hands, push a balloon with two hands, and hold an empty cardboard wrapping-paper roll with two hands to swing it. Correct her immediately if a two-handed device is swung with only one hand (such as a baseball bat).

- Involve your child in simple household activities, like wiping tables with sponges, mixing, drying dishes, and carrying trays and bins. Make sure your child uses both hands when engaging in the activity. More specific activities include using a rolling pin or sanding blocks, sweeping, raking, peeling, and grating.
- When a child struggles with reaching across the midline and rotating her trunk enough to have well-coordinated responses for bilateral activities, go back to floor play, no matter what the age. Rolling and reaching across the midline while engaged in play will help develop the necessary muscular strength and motor patterns critical to developing bilateral proficiency.

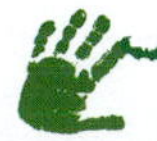

Notes

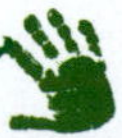

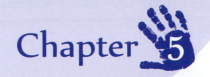

Chapter 5

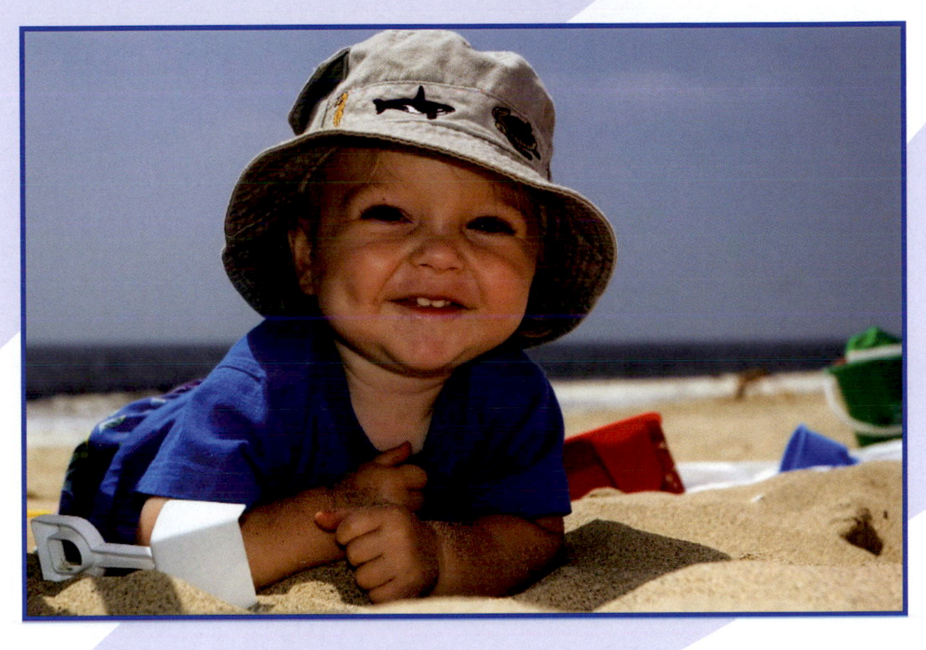

Key Motor Activities—

Toddlerhood through Grade School

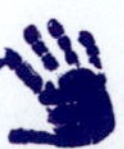

I worked with Jack for several years. Initially, he had very poor muscle tone and trunk strength, limited endurance, and poor coordination. Our work initially focused on strengthening and building his endurance. As Jack moved into kindergarten and first grade, the emphasis began to shift to coordinating his body movements. By the middle of the first grade, he learned to "pump" his body to be able to swing. At recess, Jack would charge out to the playground, making sure he reached the swings before his classmates. His teacher had never seen him run before. Jack spent the entire recess period swinging. The pumping motion helped his body get "in sync," build strength and endurance, and improve his overall coordination. His motor abilities grew exponentially from that point on. Many years later, I read in the local newspaper that Jack was on the varsity football team in high school!

Let's look at specific activities that enhance motor development. Now that your toddler has grown strong, with a flexible body and developing balance, he is ready for new challenges. Novel activities should be incorporated into his daily routine to ensure continued development of motor skills and sensorimotor integration. Certain activities are especially good for building skill sets that lay the groundwork for success in future athletic endeavors.

We'll start with swinging, because it develops isolated movement, sequencing, and a sense of rhythm while providing sensory input that is organizing to your child. Throwing and catching a ball lead to success with many eye-hand activities, whether it's catching a baseball, swinging a tennis racquet, or cradling a lacrosse stick. Riding a bike organizes the body with dynamic balancing demands, which support any activity that requires balancing (can you think of one that doesn't?). Continued development of bilateral reciprocal coordination also occurs with cycling. (The cardiovascular benefits of cycling and substituting a two-wheeled vehicle for the four-wheeled gas-guzzler are simply a collateral benefit.) Besides having the obvious value of potentially saving your child's life, swimming also continues the integration of body awareness and using both sides of the body in a coordinated way. As with cycling, cardiovascular and social benefits are also a plus.

We'll go over some tips to help teach your child these key activities as he grows. By helping your child develop these motor-skill sets, the foundations for many athletic endeavors develop.

Swinging

Many parents have used infant swings as a lifeline to prepare dinner or simply experience a few moments of peace. The swing provides a motion that usually soothes a baby's neurological system. When placed in a secure and comfortable position, this back-and-forth motion helps calm an infant. For the toddler, baby playground swings provide new sensations. The swinging motion becomes less predictable, increasing the arousal level of the child. As a toddler soars through the air, visual scenes fly back and forth as the visual system is confronted with moving stimuli. The child learns to reconcile movement with the seemingly mobile visual field.

At this point, a child's trunk does very little work. Mostly, the child learns to enjoy this new sensation of moving. Holding his head upright does activate and strengthen the neck muscles. Sometimes the child holds onto the ropes of the swing, which strengthens his hand muscles. The main accomplishment for the toddler, however, is learning to enjoy the sensation of moving with his feet off the ground.

Swinging also provides an opportunity for interaction. Wave each time your child swings toward you. This grabs your child's attention. Tell him to wave back. Engagement and interaction increase tenfold! This simple game combines language and action. As your child grows, add new challenges, such as a balloon or ball. Have him "bop the balloon" as he swings. This adds yet another dimension of planning.

When I use a swing during treatment sessions, I stand in front of the child and ask him to lift his legs into the air. Sometimes I need to help lift and straighten his little limbs. Once his legs are up in the air, I playfully grab both ankles and pull the child back and forth a few times before letting go. Each time he swings back in my direction, his legs must lift again. He is required to lift his legs each time another push is desired. Toddlers haven't learned to pump yet, but the muscles required for pumping are activated each time their legs extend.

By standing in front of your child rather than pushing from behind, the swinging becomes an active rather than a passive activity. His feet can be pushed, so his leg muscles are used. A cause-and-effect loop is established. If your child wants to go

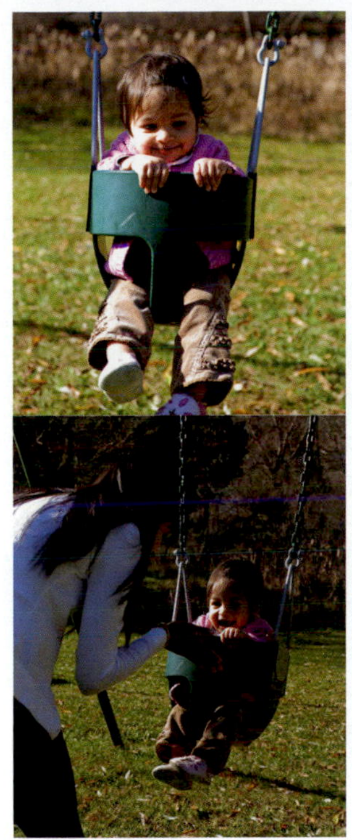

Figure 72. (a) The job of the toddler is to hold on and get used to the sensation of swinging through the air. **(b)** The opportunity for more engagement, eye contact, and language occurs when you stand in front of your toddler as you push the swing.

higher, his legs need to help facilitate this. Lifting his legs strengthens his muscles and activates the motor response required in his legs for pumping.

Swinging is identified as an important skill set because of the many aspects involved in pumping. To begin with, your child must be able to hold onto the ropes of the swing tightly. His body must be strong enough to maintain an upright position while in rapid motion. He needs to sequence several motor actions. His arms, legs, and trunk need to move individually. His arms pull and push, while his legs flex and straighten. His trunk bends backward and forward at the waist in coordination with the other movements. These sequenced movements need to be timed perfectly. Rather than attempting to parse this phenomenon, suffice it to say that swinging is complicated!

The motor lessons learned from the swinging sequence are many. Your child learns to respond to the swinging motion in a coordinated way. The reciprocal movement of the arms and legs must follow a pattern, just as dance steps follow a certain sequence. The smoother the execution of this motor sequence, the higher and faster your child will swing. When an incorrect sequence is applied, the swinging motion slows or stops altogether.

While it's initially difficult to get in sync with this sequence, once it's established, the motion is rhythmic and helps establish a sense of rhythm within the body. The movement requires core strength, which develops endurance in the trunk and limbs. The sensation of swinging can be a very organizing one. It may calm and help focus your child, and this focus carries over to other activities when the swinging session is over. Once your child masters swinging, it frequently becomes a favorite activity.

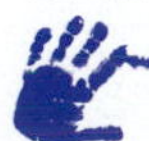

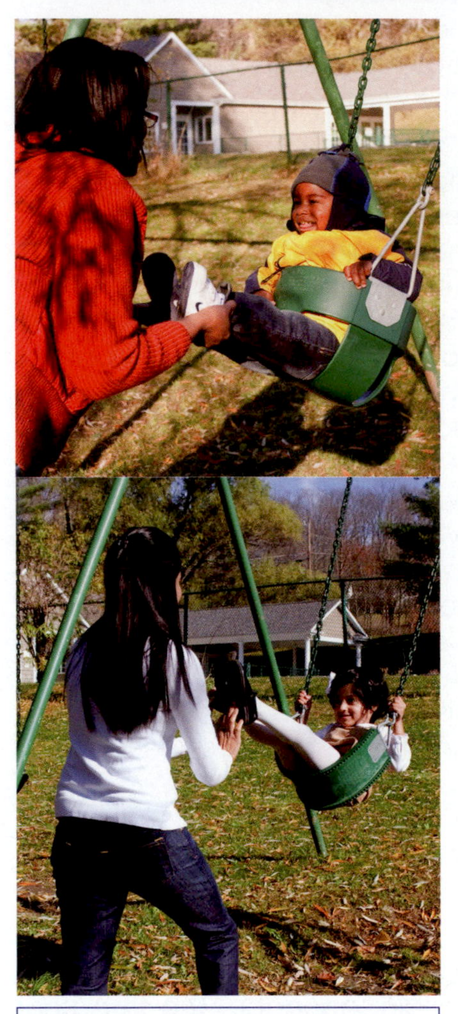

Figure 73. (a) By grabbing the legs of an older toddler, the activity becomes more dynamic. Creating rapid, stop-and-go motions and encouraging verbal responses, such as "Are you ready?" and "Ready, set, go!" make the activity more interactive, fun, and integrating as the child manages the motor challenges of swinging coupled with simple language demands. **(b)** For the preschooler, the child must lift and extend her legs for each push. This facilitates the correct motor sequence for pumping.

Do not underestimate the exercise required and the benefits reaped from swinging. I worked with an older child, Charlie, who struggled to learn how to pump. Limited trunk strength and motor-planning difficulties made many activities very difficult for him. Once Charlie learned to pump on the swing, he was encouraged to swing every day, for all of the benefits listed earlier. Unfortunately, with his extra body weight and poor physical endurance, this was akin to demanding an hour of push-ups and abdominal crunches. To build his endurance, during therapy, I required him to pump the swing 100 times while we counted. Charlie considered me his personal torturer during these sessions.

Fortunately, for most children, once the skill of swinging is mastered, many hours a day can be spent in the backyard or on the playground, pumping the swing. An adult no longer needs to intervene, thereby giving the child time to experience independence and mastery over his little body **(Figures 72 and 73)**.

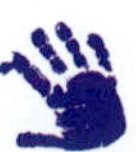

Recommended Activities

- Engage your child in swinging at an early age. This helps your baby become familiar and comfortable with this type of motion. With a younger child, make sure there is adequate support for his trunk and head. The speed should be regulated by what the child can tolerate. If his body is flopping around, more support may be necessary, and the speed of swinging may be too fast.
- Make swinging interactive - wave or say "hi" each time your child approaches. Push your baby from the front, so he can see your face.
- As your toddler progresses, ask him to lift his legs so pushing occurs in his feet. This establishes one of the movements for pumping, strengthens his legs, and engages him in the process physically.
- Once your child moves to a regular, unsupported swing, continue with the extended legs for pushing. Suggest that your child lean back and pull on the ropes at the same time.
- Once this movement is established, tell your child to bend his legs immediately after his feet are pushed. His trunk may begin to lean forward, and his arms should push against the ropes.
- Repeating a "push-pull" mantra might help get your child in sync with the movements.
- If your child struggles with the motor sequence, have him sit on your lap while you swing, so he can feel the movement and rhythm required. Coupling words with the movements helps, as well.
- Teeter-totters or gliders help establish the pushing and pulling motor sequence. Opportunities to ride on these help your child learn the basic mechanics necessary for pumping.
- Remember, your child must be developmentally ready to pump independently. The trunk must be strong, and the arms and legs should move separately. When children can skip, they are ready to pump on a swing.

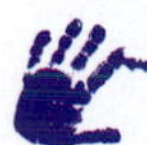

Throwing and Catching a Ball

When people discuss eye-hand coordination, throwing and catching a ball are often the first things that come to mind. They are quintessential uses of the eye-hand connection. As such, learning to throw and catch establishes a very important base for all activities involving eye-hand coordination in the larger motor arena. Someone who has pitched for a professional baseball team will likely have a very fast tennis serve. The person's accuracy might need tweaking, but the ability to rotate the arm and snap the wrist are highly developed and transfer easily to serving a tennis ball. Visually following a slowly rolled or tossed ball leads to eventual success with a speeding puck or a bouncing basketball.

Eye-hand coordination begins moments after birth. As an infant's eyes open and focus on his or her caretaker, this developmental process begins. In the nursery, a baby's eyes follow sounds and peripheral motions. Engaging the baby by jingling objects, such as keys and rattles, and moving them slowly back and forth leads to the development of visual tracking.

When a baby swats at a hanging toy intentionally (with or without a celebratory mariachi band), the eye-hand connection begins. The infant sees an interesting object and moves her hand with an intent to touch and explore it. Early in life, these experiences should be duplicated over and over again. Encouraging your baby to observe and then reach for an interesting toy leads to a connection between the eyes and hands working together. Eyes and hands become team players; one requires the other to complete the job.

During my oldest son's first year of life, I commuted to New York several days a week. The trip took 2 hours each way, barring traffic. While Chris waited for his mom (and dinner!) to arrive, his dad would stack several wooden blocks on the floor and wait for Chris to knock them over. This was done repeatedly and with great delight. My husband placed the blocks in various locations, challenging Chris to reach farther and in different directions. Along with successfully distracting him from the long wait to see Mommy, Chris was developing a good sense of how his arm needed to move to achieve his goal.

Even when a baby is still lying on her tummy for playtime, rolling a ball to her initiates directed eye-hand play. Knocking over stacked blocks, pushing a toy truck, and throwing Cheerios off the high-chair tray all provide opportunities for a baby to experiment with the cause-and-effect of hands and eyes working together.

The actual throw-and-catch motion begins in earnest with modified movements, such as rolling the ball.

Here's a typical sequence of ball play:

- A ball is rolled to the baby. The baby reaches out to grab it. Uncoordinated batting of the ball to send it back may occur. Usually without initial success.
- The ball is rolled back and forth successfully.
- Primitive throwing occurs, usually underhand or sideways in first attempts.
- At 3 years old, overhead throwing should occur for short distances.
- Early catching begins with the child's arms fully extended, waiting for the ball to land directly in her open arms. Her arms then hug ball into her chest to secure it.
- Her arms gradually bend, and the ball is caught in her open hands. At 4 years old, the child stops trapping the ball into her chest. At 6 years old, she can catch a tennis ball in her hands.
- At 4 years old, overhead throwing occurs for longer distances (10 feet and more).
- Bouncing and catching a bounced ball occur somewhere in the 4- to 5-year-old range.

Specific games can be played to help facilitate the development of throwing and catching. As mentioned earlier, rolling a ball helps activate visual tracking and the eye-hand connection. Speeding up the rolling game and rolling the ball in slightly different directions teaches her eyes to track faster and anticipate new movement. In essence, it helps establish flexibility in the visual-motor system.

When playing fetch, a well-trained dog will watch its owner closely until the stick is thrown; a less disciplined dog will enthu-

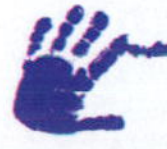

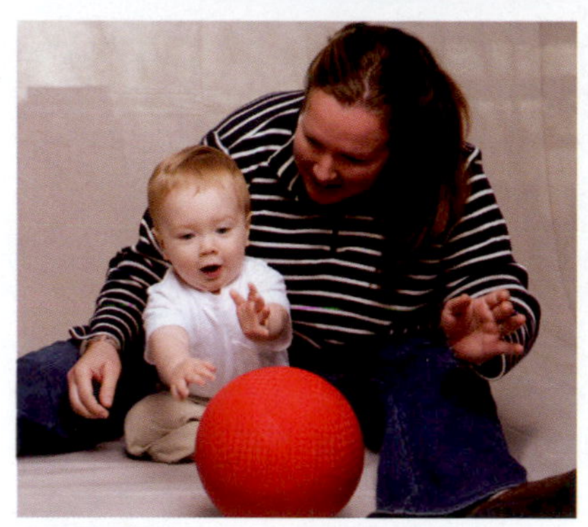

Figure 74. Learning to catch and throw a ball. To establish a base for catching, begin rolling balls and other slow-moving objects, such as balloons, beanbags, beach balls, Gertie balls, and Kooshes to your child.

siastically run in the direction of a previously thrown stick, missing the point of looking at the stick as it is thrown to determine its destination. Likewise, children need to pay attention to the movement of an object, not guess on the basis of previous experience.

Initially, show and perhaps help your baby feel how to move her arms to push the ball away. While pushing a ball seems like one simple step, it actually requires the linking of several motor demands. The child must follow the ball with her eyes, get her arms and hands ready, then move them to make contact with the ball. Finally, she needs to learn to keep moving her arms after contact is made, to complete the follow-through that propels the ball forward.

Babies generally have ample opportunities to practice throwing. They throw their stuffed animals, food, plastic toys, and anything else available. Besides moving their arms, throwing also requires timing in the release of the object. Professional pitchers have the release of a ball down to a science. The wrist is held at an exact angle, and release occurs at a specific moment to deliver a slider, a curveball, or a fastball. Young children use a trial-and-error process to figure out the best way to heave an object. Repetition is key. The object might be anything that happens to be within reach at any given moment.

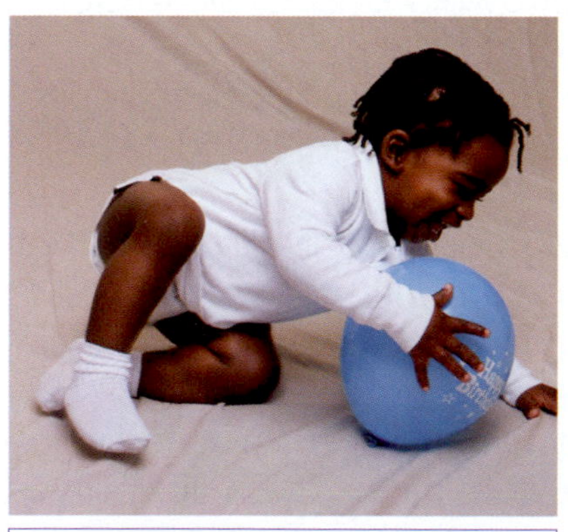

Figure 75. Wayne enjoys retrieving this balloon.

Young children are frequently caught throwing sticks and stones. Generally, the intent has nothing to do with hurting someone. It has everything to do with practicing this primary and very important movement. Just as a

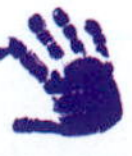

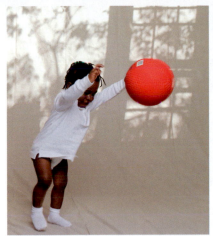

Figure 76. Early throwing begins with flinging the ball up into the air with two hands. The whole body moves as a unit. This segues into a side-arm toss, where the entire arm is straight like a stick. By continuing to use a large ball, as Wayne does here, a child must use two hands, forcing rotation in the trunk as the transition to a sideways toss begins. This helps strengthen the lateral muscles that are so important later on when the pitcher winds up to throw that curveball.

young swinger will pump his legs for hours on the playground, a neophyte thrower will execute the throwing motion repeatedly until the task is mastered **(Figures 74-76)**.

Playing "tossing" games helps satisfy the craving to throw objects and channel the motion into a goal-directed activity. Beanbag tosses, Velcro dartboards, and simply tossing designated "safe" toys toward a target, such as a basket or cardboard box, all provide healthy outlets for a young "pitcher." Varying the objects and targets provides novelty, which piques a child's interest and engagement.

Toddlers and preschoolers will endure throwing and catching practice or "drills" with Uncle Willie in the backyard because they yearn for the opportunity to spend uninterrupted time with a beloved family member. The enjoyment of quality time with a loved one is usually the primary motivator as to why a child sticks with a task. The inherent value of the "skill training" is lost on a child. This doesn't mean family members and caretakers should stop playing catch in the yard. Simply recognize that a young child needs variety and has a short attention span. The love and affection of a significant other is far more important to a child than any long-term goal of becoming a star athlete.

Recommended Activities

- Engage in opportunities for your baby to look at and follow interesting visual stimuli every day, from birth onward.
- Have your baby reach out and grasp a variety of objects, beginning with your finger, soon after birth.
- Interacting with sensory-rich objects (with bright colors, varied textures, and sounds) enhances your child's manipulative and visual experiences as she grows.
- When your child's hands begin to bat at and grasp things independently, provide opportunities throughout the day for looking, reaching, and grasping.
- Suspended mobiles have some value, but this is limited. Initial exposure may spark your child's interest, but then it wanes. Just as an adult enjoys a visual image and then moves on, a baby needs dynamic visual information to sustain her attention.
- Dynamic interaction with another human being remains the ideal visual stimulus. Siblings holding a favorite toy in front of the baby's face, a grandparent playing peek-a-boo, and the babysitter holding objects for the infant to bat at all provide experiences that lead to active engagement.
- As reaching improves, set up play scenarios that create cause-and-effect experiences. Knocking over a stack of blocks, pressing a button to make a toy move, and pushing a toy truck are activities that improve a baby's eye-hand connectivity.
- Introduction to ball play should occur with rolling the ball. This is slow and predictable. Gradually increase the speed and vary the direction of the movement (roll it to the left side and then the right side of the toddler).
- Catching a ball should be introduced by using a medium-sized soft ball (6-10 inches in diameter), such as a foam or cloth ball. An inverse relationship related to the size and speed of the ball should occur as the child's proficiency improves (with practice, a smaller

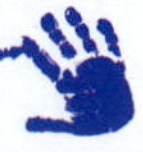

ball can be introduced and rolled or thrown at a faster pace).

- Here's the typical progression of learning to catch:
    - The child has rigid, straight arms with open hands and will trap the ball to her chest to catch it by 3 years old.
    - The child has slightly bent arms and will still trap the ball to her chest.
    - The child has bent, flexible arms and will catch the ball in her hands by 4 years of age.
    - The child learns to catch the ball with one hand by 6 years of age.
- If your child closes her eyes as the ball approaches her, play a game with balloons, in which the balloon is bopped gently on her face. This allows her to become less fearful of an object moving quickly toward her face. With reduced fears, the child will learn not to look away and will be better able to track the ball.
- Overhead throwing can be introduced around 3 years old, but real drill-type work should not occur until 4 to 6 years old. Keep in mind that a 4-year-old's attention span remains quite short, so throwing sessions should be limited and brief. Try to mix running around and horseplay with these practice sessions.

Riding a Bicycle

Riding a bike is like toilet training. You, as a parent, cannot control the process. Your child will not allow you to let go until her confidence develops. Until that moment, no matter how prepared you feel your child is to ride independently, she will insist on having your support. As a "coach," you can do everything necessary to help your child learn, but the actual "letting go," figuratively and otherwise, comes from your child. With toilet training, it is a question of autonomy and having control of one's bodily functions. With cycling, it is the sense of confidence that the body will meet the challenge of maintaining balance and

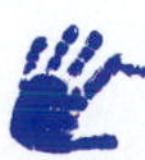

protecting oneself if a fall occurs. Both are scary and powerful.

There are many adults who have never ridden a bike or have put the bike away for life, with no intention of getting on it again. So, you may ask, why is cycling a key activity for overall motor development?

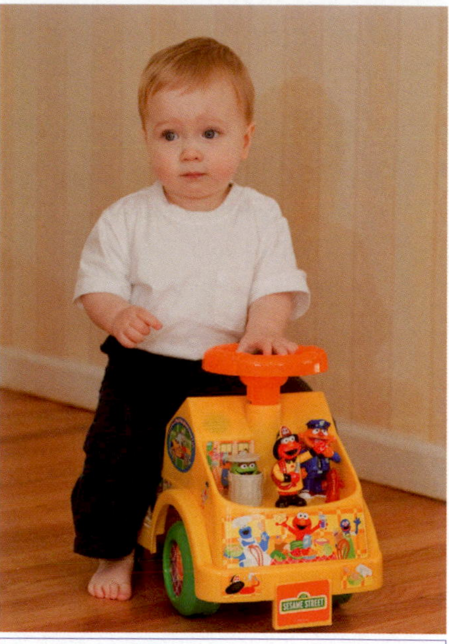

Figure 77. Little ride-on toys accustom your child to the sensation of moving while straddling a toy. The toddler's legs learn to move together in a bilateral pattern, where they execute the same movement at the same time. Riding a tricycle helps a preschooler learn to pedal and steer.

Riding a bicycle presents motor challenges that no other athletic activity offers. It requires the ability to maintain balance with your feet off the ground. This balance needs to be maintained while speeding up and slowing down. It necessitates the ability to operate a piece of equipment (the bicycle) in coordination with the body. This involves timing, spatial awareness, and planning. The mechanics of riding a bicycle include reciprocal movements of the legs for spinning the pedals and dynamic balancing. It also requires the use of the arms and hands to steer. The entire body must be engaged at all times. The eyes must be vigilant in guiding the bicycle. All these components are necessary to develop the skill of riding a bike.

Balance. Your child will not allow you to "let go" of the bike until a sense of balance, albeit wobbly, is attained. Balancing on a bike is not the same as standing on one foot. It is balance that occurs as the body moves. This requires the activation of many trunk muscles throughout the body.

For most skiers, even those in excellent physical condition, after the first day on the slopes, muscles ache throughout the body. This is because the dynamic balancing required for skiing activates deep muscles that maintain a person's center of gravity. The demands of flying down the slopes, avoiding near falls, and shifting the body from side to side while turning require

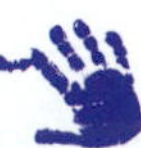

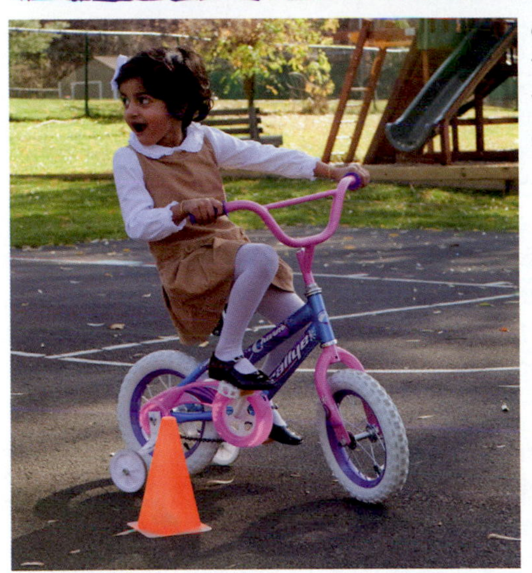

Figure 78. Setting up courses on the playground helps refine steering ability and increases directional sense. When making the big jump to a two-wheeler, make sure your child has learned how to safely stop herself from falling by extending her leg(s). A small bike, from which her feet can comfortably touch the ground, is essential.

all the muscles in the body to move in different ways than they do for walking and running.

Likewise, when cycling, these muscles must be ready for action. If your child has engaged in lots of floor time, climbing, rolling, and all the other good forms of play discussed earlier in the book, the little muscles throughout his body that are necessary for dynamic balancing and solid trunk control should be ready for action. These muscles will be ready for the work of riding a bike.

Reciprocal movement of the legs. Remember the cruising baby, holding onto a ledge while his foot shifted sideways? One leg moved, followed by the other. Gradually, the cruising pattern improved. This sideways walk developed a pattern and rhythm that readied the child for the reciprocal movement of walking. Looking back even further, crawling in four-point position provided a wonderful opportunity for the child's legs to move reciprocally. Ease in motor sequencing facilitates ease in pedaling.

Cycling requires an alternating motion of the legs. One leg pushes the pedal down, as the other lifts or pulls up. The rotating crank helps to regulate the motion, but the child must be able to execute the push-pull-lift movement repetitively. Toddlers begin with ride-on toys that have no pedals attached. Their feet push and pull the toy forward on the floor. The legs work in unison, making the same movement at the same time. Moving on to a tricycle is a big step. To be able to move the tricycle, pedaling must occur. Each leg must push down one pedal at a time. The child must be coordinated and strong enough to push down with one leg while the other leg lifts up. Each foot must stay firmly on

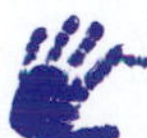

top of the pedal while it rotates around the crank axis **(Figure 77)**.

Guidance from the eyes. As a child learns to pedal, his eyes need to move from his legs to the path in which the tricycle or bicycle is traveling. This requires a good sense of where his legs are positioned (is his foot resting securely on the pedal?). It also requires an awareness of how his legs are moving and the ability to pay attention to both legs at the same time. With good body awareness in place, the child can direct visual attention to the road and adjust the riding to the terrain, which requires the ability to steer, control speed, and anticipate conditions.

One of the reasons tricycles are so important is that they offer ample opportunities for a child to acquire rudimentary skills in pedaling and steering. Setting up little courses, such as moving around cones, gives a child such practice **(Figure 78)**. Once a child steps up to using a two-wheeler with training wheels, refinement of steering agility continues.

When your child finally rides solo on a two-wheeler, his attention may shift to the dynamics of balancing and pedaling, so the steering becomes quite wild. Beginning these early voyages in wide-open spaces allows for a significant margin of error until he begins to assimilate the other motor demands and, thus, can begin focusing on steerage again. Before you let go of the seat, have your child move around a course to practice steering. This helps solidify the mechanics of riding. Familiarity with each component minimizes missteps in the solo ride, thereby reducing the number of crashes.

Speed control mostly occurs from trial-and-error learning and practice. Early experiences of flying down a hill on a trike for the thrill of crashing or trying to turn on a tricycle too fast help teach the limitations of speed. Riding with training wheels provides the opportunity to practice starting and stopping, as well as experiment with increasing speed. Learning to regulate speed mostly requires practice and a few scraped knees. You can play "fast/slow" games that require your child to speed up and slow down on command. This helps him develop the proficiency that will be required for using the brakes with a two-wheeler.

Above all, cycling requires the determination and the opportunity to practice. Children who live on cul-de-sacs or have wide open, paved playgrounds nearby usually learn to

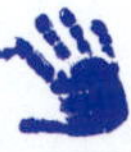

ride first. This is because they can pick up a bike, pedal a few times, fall a few times, and then quit for a while. The child can run away from the bike to play on the playground or simply rest until the courage and energy are mustered to return to the bike and try again. Sadly, in a world with fewer sidewalks and kid-friendly areas, fewer opportunities for "organically learning" to ride a bike exist. Often, learning to ride a bike requires "training sessions." You have to haul the bike into the car and drive to an open parking lot when little traffic is anticipated. A designated amount of time to practice bike-riding is scheduled. Rest periods to play on the swings or simply take a break detract from the practice time allotted, thereby making these breaks feel like wasted time. Frequently, these become stressed and frustrating exercises rather than fun-filled outings to play.

Recommended Activities

- When your child becomes a toddler, purchase or borrow an inexpensive riding toy, such as a trike. Allow your child to cruise around the house and eventually outside. Expand the challenge by making obstacle courses, so rudimentary steering concepts develop. If a safe, gently sloping terrain is available, allow your child to ride down the slope. This helps him learn how to manage speed. Relatively safe "crashing" on these low vehicles teaches important lessons in controlling the ride.
- Upright tricycles simulate the same pedaling motion used for cycling. Once again, engineer opportunities for steering and speed changes to help solidify these concepts. Avoid the same crashing scenarios the toddler enjoyed with a trike situated lower to the ground, as falling from an upright tricycle can be painful and potentially injurious.
- The same goes for training wheels. Your child rides higher off the ground, so the simulation to real cycling is a much closer approximation. Your child should become very comfortable and facile with all components of riding with training wheels before taking them off. A counter-argument is to move directly from a tricycle to a two-

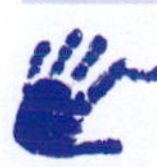

wheeler. If your child rides a tricycle as if participating in the Tour de France and is highly motivated to move on to the real deal, then by all means try a two-wheeler. However, make sure it sits low to the ground, so falls will hurt less when they happen. Keep in mind that this is essentially a "sink or swim" approach.

- A smaller two-wheeler will provide a sense of security, as your child's feet can touch the ground readily, and potential falls occur from a much lower vantage point. While his big brother's hand-me-down bike may be tempting, size is key, so you may want to ask cousins and neighbors if you can borrow a more appropriately sized bicycle.
- The first bike will be battered and bruised if it's utilized fully, so while the enthusiasm for a shiny new bike beckons to many parents, think long and hard about the implications of turning down that hand-me-down available just around the corner. A new bike will look just like the hand-me-down in a matter of days. With a used bike, the first scratch will not be as traumatizing and may even go unnoticed. Avoiding guilt early on in the parent-child relationship is a wonderful thing!
- If bike-riding practice requires a trip to a parking lot or some other bike- and kid-friendly location, consider packing a picnic lunch and make an outing out of it. That lifts the pressure off the performance aspect of the "training session" and gives the child time to regroup between rides. Running, climbing, and swinging all help "reorganize" his brain and ready your child for more action.
- With the training wheels off, practice how to stop a fall before moving one inch forward. Find a curb, and position the bicycle parallel to it. Have your child sit on the seat and rest one foot on the curb for balance. His other foot should rest on the pedal. Gently tip the bike away from the curb. Your child will quickly lift his foot off the pedal and place it on the ground to stop himself from falling. This should be repeated many times (like 100!) and then duplicated in the opposite

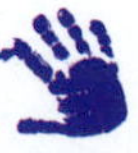

direction. Once your child has an understanding of how to fall safely and an automatic response has been established, he will have more confidence with moving forward.

- Continue with curb training. Have your child propel himself forward with his curbside foot, as if he's using a scooter. He should allow his other foot to passively ride the pedal. Occasionally, have your child lift both feet up to experience the gliding motion and the feel of basic balancing.
- Now begins the exciting part. Your child mounts the saddle, while you stabilize the bicycle. Have your child pedal slowly while you steady the bike. As the momentum increases, the forward motion should help center the bike. If stability appears fairly well established, let go, but be ready to run and catch a falling vehicle. If met with initial failure, try, try again. If no forward progress is made, go back to the curb. If this is too hard, go back to floor play and trunk strengthening!
- Negotiation and trust are an integral part of this process. Discuss with your neophyte cyclist how much support you will give and when you will pull back. You are a team, and communication is key. Motivating and building confidence in your young rider is often the most important part of the process. Continue the dance of supporting and letting go until your child safely rides off into the sunset.

Swimming

Swimming provides motor challenges similar to those of cycling—reciprocal arm and leg movements coordinated with movements of the head and neck for breathing. It builds strength and endurance, especially in the trunk muscles, which are so important for general conditioning and overall health. Unlike other sports, however, *being able to swim can make all the difference between life and death.*

Knowing how to swim ripples out to the next generation. Parents who can swim tend to relax and enjoy the water. This imparts a sense of fun related to water play and eventual

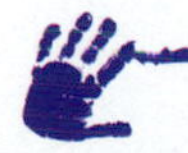

swimming. Nonswimmers usually convey anxiety to their children, no matter how carefully they try to hide it while in the water. Children are extremely perceptive and quickly pick up on this tension. Why would they want to play in this strange substance when fear is so palpable? When a child learns to swim, the cycle of fear ends, and these insecurities are no longer passed on to the next generation.

Life versus death is a stand-alone reason for all human beings to learn to swim. But there are actually many other compelling reasons to consider swimming as a high priority. For a child, it develops many great benefits in terms of gross-motor abilities and general physical conditioning. Swimming also opens up social venues for a child. A youngster who can jump safely and with abandon into the deep end of the pool has a much better time at a pool party—guaranteed—than a child who is waiting for the "swimmies" to be affixed. Positive engagement in the water carries over to having fun at class picnics and beyond.

Besides the fun, swimming provides a sense of accomplishment of extreme proportions **(Figure 79)**. Learning to float (a.k.a. "not sink") defies the threat that water poses. Mastering underwater swimming, such as being able to retrieve a toy from the bottom of the pool, takes a child into territory that was previously off-limits. Traversing the length of the pool requires endurance, skill, and courage.

To raise a successful swimmer, encourage water play from infancy onward. Splashing in the tub during bath time should be a joyful time rather than a stressful one.

Baby water classes are available and offer many approaches to introducing your infant to the water. Reviewing those programs is not in the scope of this book. However, if air and water temperatures permit, hold your baby while moving gently through the water, with her head held securely above the surface. Sing or talk to her as you introduce her to the water to make it a fun and soothing experience.

There are many approaches to teaching your child to swim. The two key ingredients are the following. First, your child must learn to be unafraid. Second, your child needs to learn how to hold her breath underwater. Skills such as floating will progress naturally if your child learns to relax while in the water.

Learning to submerge her head can begin in the tub. Tipping her chin and mouth into the water to blow bubbles, like a motorboat, is step number one. Tipping her whole face in while holding her breath is step two. Having a washcloth at the ready to wipe off the water if necessary might help.

Once your child can safely hold her breath when submerged, family play in the water can begin. Hold your child close and bob up and down, submerging more of her body each time. Eventually, bob down so that her head begins to go slightly under the surface. Repeat this with increasing depth. Laughter with each dunk and exclamations of glee should correspond with this activity. Cues such as "Are you ready!?" and exaggerating the inhalation and breath-holding can precede the dunking. If your child is not sharing in the joy, go back to less threatening water play.

Another avenue to submersion occurs in gently sloping water depths. Placing toys on the bottom of the pool for your child to pick up eventually leads to a need to reach down so far that her head goes beneath the surface of the water to retrieve the toys. Your child will self-regulate this process. The toy will not be obtained until she feels confident about submerging her head to reach it.

Once holding her breath and enjoying the water are established, swim lessons, either formal or informal, should proceed without problems. You should determine if your child prefers instruction from new individuals or someone familiar. Some do better following directions from a designated authority figure, such as an instructor, instead of a parent. Others remain shy around strangers and prefer home teaching.

If you are fearful of the water as a parent, consider enlisting a friend or relative to be your child's "swimming coach." Avoid infecting your child with anxiety about being in the water. It is difficult to cure once acquired!

Do not scoff at those little blow-up wading pools, which can be purchased at the five-and-dime for less than 30 dollars. Little wading pools provide opportunities for exploration at your child's own pace, rather than the pace of a swim class or your agenda as a parent. Like riding a bike, the opportunity to try out some of the developing skills without any pressure or demands

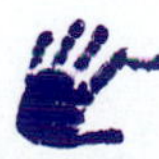

from you as a parent help your child to gain confidence. Swim time needs to be supervised closely, particularly in pools, ponds, and larger bodies of water, as your child's safety is paramount. In these more treacherous environments, a child's opportunities to self-explore are somewhat limited. In a small pool that's only 6 to 8 inches deep, supervision is still necessary, but your child has more freedom to move around and try out simple things, such as ducking under the water to retrieve a toy, when the courage is finally mustered. At 8 inches, your child feels safe in that no unseen terrors are lurking beneath the surface, and the distance seems fairly manageable so that reemerging from the shallow depth is a pretty good bet. In shallow water, your child can also "pretend swim" by positioning her body downward and mocking swim strokes with her hands pushing off the bottom, while holding her body up. Over time, this may lead to the sensation of floating and certainly begins to lay the foundation for the motor plan of swimming.

And the List Goes on...

There are many other sports that offer specific skills and benefits beyond this basic list. Soccer establishes eye-foot coordination and develops legwork, which transfers to other sports easily. Tumbling and gymnastics develop body awareness, positioning in space, and moving in more sophisticated ways, as well as teaching the body how to orient and move while upside down and airborne.

Martial arts and dancing train the body to move in a controlled and balanced way, as well as develop skills with complicated sequenced movements. "Stick" sports, such as tennis, hockey, lacrosse, golf, and baseball, all extend and challenge eye-hand coordination skills to new limits. Basketball synthesizes the ball-handling skills of bouncing, throwing, and catching with the demand of responding to others. Horseback riding introduces an element beyond cycling, managing not only a moving object but also a living one with a will of its own.

Any and all sports provide opportunities for your child's body to become stronger and more coordinated. They enhance overall body awareness and corresponding comfort

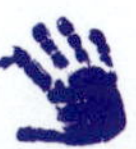

with living "in one's own skin." Team sports develop an ability to play with others, learn rules, negotiate, and develop specific game skills. Your child also learns to organize movements to respond to the frequently unpredictable movements of others. Training builds endurance. Setting goals and achieving them helps your child learn that many barriers are artificial and are made to be broken. These lessons often flow into other life experiences, making your child more adaptable, tenacious, and persevering.

Positive benefits abound when athletic endeavors occur in a balanced and healthy way. As has been stressed throughout this book, your child must be developmentally ready for each new step in motor training. Pushing a child before the physical or emotional readiness occurs leads to a sense of failure, frustration, and/or resentment and lack of confidence. The potential love of a sport may be lost. Allow your child to take the lead or at least collaborate in the decision-making process of which sport(s) to choose and how frequently to participate.

Recommended Activities

- Learning basic motor skills should be a joyful process for both you and your child. If an activity matches the maturity level of your child, and realistic expectations are made regarding attention span and energy level, a good time should be had by all.
- Sandwich fledgling skills in between activities that have been mastered so that your child begins with a sense of success and ends with a sense of accomplishment, no matter how difficult the target challenge might be. Make sure to have free and silly play wrapped around any practice time. Roughhousing is always a welcome and helpful way to enhance body awareness without any planned motor demands.
- Choosing which sport(s) to pursue should be a child-driven decision. Family members obviously influence this process via exposure to various sports. Some children prefer to try out many different activities over the course of several years. Others focus on one or two. Some children prefer to keep the play unstructured and delay entrance into

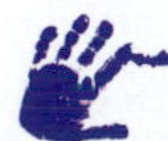

the sports arena until later in development.

- How do you know when your child is ready to increase the intensity of training and commitment to one sport? Look and listen to your child. Does he appear enthusiastic? Or does he hang back or appear unhappy after games and practice? Often, having a discussion with a coach can help you get a read on your child's readiness. Weigh the pros and cons with your child, as well.
- When entering the formal athletic arena, whether it is soccer, Little League, hockey, or dance, the most important factor in your child's success and enjoyment relates to the coaches' understanding of development. Before placing your child on a team or in a class, it is important to determine if the instructor understands the importance of motor, social, and emotional development. If the coach talks a lot about how many "championship seasons" he or she has had and talks very little about the individual needs of each child, look for another team.
- Good coaching combines an understanding of development with the appropriate skills to be taught. All skills should be developed in each player. Specialization too early in development stunts the overall athletic development of a young athlete.

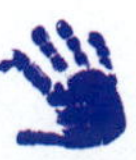

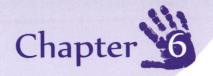

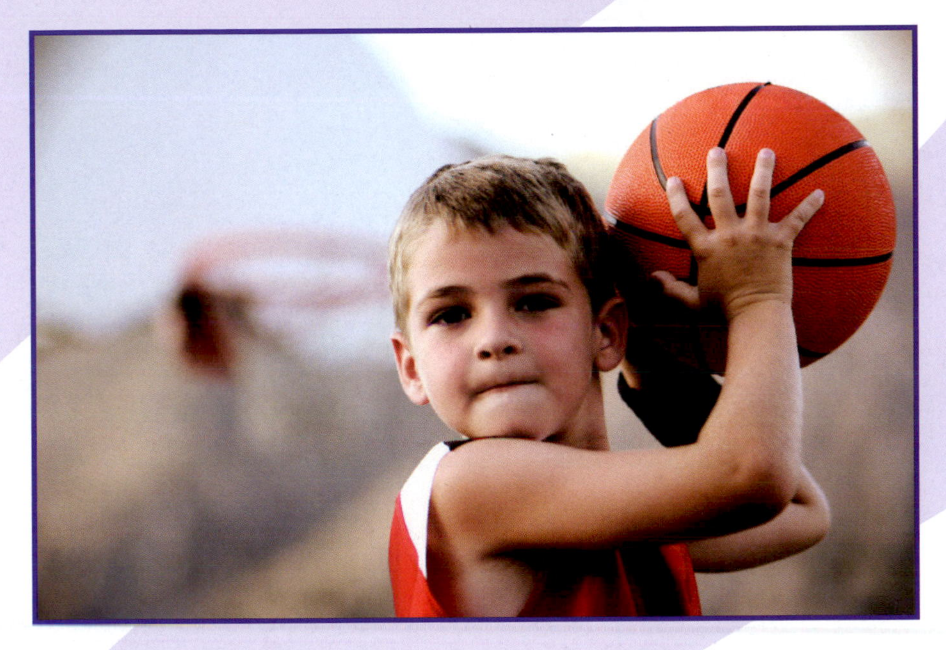

Introducing Formal Sports

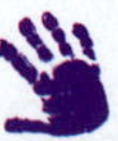

Your growing child has learned the lessons of motor development so well that you now feel terror on the playground as your child seeks out new challenges. If your child has begun to remind you of Evel Knieval, executing hair-raising jumps on a bike and engaging in other spine-chilling activities, it might be time to ramp up the motor challenges in his life! At some point, it becomes apparent that this growing motor machine needs new activities to test his growing physical prowess.

This chapter looks at the many factors to consider when determining the right time to introduce formal athletics. Which sport to play or how many sports to try comes into question. How to select the "right" activity and what level of intensity to choose all become important questions in balancing your child's growing appetite for motor challenges and the need to keep your child's world "sane."

Several motor activities were outlined in the last chapter to illustrate the benefits to overall motor development. The next logical step for some children is to pursue a specific sport. Parents often ask questions regarding the introduction of sports into their child's life. How early? Which sport is best? How many? Obviously, your child should be a large player in making this decision, as there are many considerations involved:

- Developmental readiness of the child. This includes emotional and social readiness, as well as physical strength and coordination.
- Availability of developmentally appropriate instruction and coaching.
- The child's (as well as the family's) expressed interest.
- Weighing the value of unstructured playtime against structured, adult-driven activities.

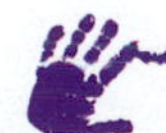

Developmental Readiness

Many aspects of motor development contribute to a child's overall physical health and success in motor activities. When determining whether your child is ready to enroll in a structured sport, the following components come into play:

1. Does my child have adequate strength and endurance, given the amount of time required for the specified activity?

If your child gets fatigued by walking across the parking lot and wants to be held during each visit to the grocery store, the demand of running around a field for 60 minutes might be unrealistic.

If your child always chooses sedentary activities, such as sand play at the park, and needs a great deal of encouragement to join other children (possibly even withdrawing frequently and refusing to participate), asking your child to garner the stamina to play with a team may be asking too much.

While the hope may be that participating in a team sport will increase her strength and build endurance, the child needs to meet baseline criteria (for example, being comfortable with running around for 30 minutes). If your child has never run around for more than 5 minutes at a time without pooping out, and the intended practice time is 60 minutes, this scenario may lead to your child experiencing a sense of failure, and you as a parent will likely have a very frustrating experience.

2. Does my child have the motor-planning skills necessary to engage successfully in this particular sport?

If your child gets confused in large groups and has a difficult time understanding what to do, the demands of team instruction might be difficult.

If your child consistently understands and learns with one-on-one instruction, but confusion and frustration ensue when he's taught in a large group, joining a team might be premature.

You may observe your child standing passively in the sporting arena, maybe even with a stubborn or uncooperative appearance. Usually, he is simply overwhelmed and confused.

Some children run around impulsively, doing all kinds of tricks but not doing specifically what's been requested. Frequently,

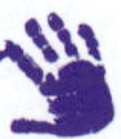

when a child cannot figure out how to execute the specified motor action, a process of trial and error occurs. Similar to the student who isn't sure how to answer an essay question, so he writes down everything he knows on the subject, a child with motor-planning difficulties will move in a multitude of ways, hoping that one of the actions will match what the instructor has told the group to do.

In a carefully selected environment, structured activities may be an excellent way for your child to acquire motor skills and build motor-planning abilities. It is important, however, to conduct a careful assessment of the group dynamics and your child's ability to carry out instructions and replicate the motor demands requested.

With both physical stamina and motor-planning ability, it is important to match your child's readiness level with the activity. Studies have shown that "when children feel that they will not be able to perform adequately to the performance demands of the competition, they experience [a] threat to self-esteem, which results in stress."[3]

3. Can my child manage the sensory demands of the surrounding environment?

At birthday parties, some children run around, getting more and more wound up until they practically explode. Excitement quickly leads to disorganized behavior. Others hate attending parties, and they cover their ears to block out all the noise. They often need to be encouraged by an adult to participate. If your child gets excited easily and has difficulty organizing subsequent behaviors, the dynamic nature of team sports may be too much.

My husband coached "G Patrol," the entry-level soccer event otherwise known as "Swarm Ball." The main objective of this team experience is to introduce children to the concept of kicking a ball, running, and playing with other children. While this was a purely recreational experience, with no pressure to "perform," the way children on the team reacted to this neophyte experience ran the gamut. Some moved around the field with abandon, kicking the ball or following the "scrum" as they obliviously crossed the designated playing field and beyond. Other children became overwhelmed or confused and ran off the field into the arms of Mom or Dad. With

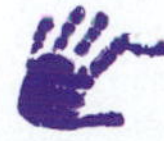

encouragement, many dried their tears, ran back onto the field, and learned to love the experience. For others, standing next to Mom or hugging Dad's leg was where they wanted to be. Years later, one of the "leg huggers" wound up attending West Point. Was there a motor deficiency? Absolutely not. The little boy simply wasn't ready to jump into the athletic arena just yet. His parents respected this. Clearly, when he was ready, he did quite well in the athletic realm.

In a situation such as this, observe the surrounding environment, the way the coaching occurs, and how the children interact and move around. These clues will indicate to you whether your child will manage the environment and thrive in it. If the environment is too loud or too busy, the child's enjoyment and ability to perform may be impeded. Feeling a basic level of comfort with the surroundings is necessary for a child to be able to organize the learning of new behaviors, such as catching a ball or doing an arabesque.

4. Social and emotional readiness is key in having a successful experience with a structured group activity.

Your child may be as strong as a tank and incredibly coordinated but wails every time he is separated from Mommy. Asking a child like this to leave his safety zone of Mom and his home and venture into the strange territory of a playing field, gym, or studio may be too much.

Some children get very excited whenever they visit a friend. This excitement may lead to hugging the friend too roughly and too often. This behavior indicates that the child has not learned the concept and importance of personal space. This overzealousness becomes a challenge for the child to overcome, as playmates do not appreciate infringements of their personal space. As children attempt to engage in new athletic endeavors, this tendency can become problematic.

Some children are fiercely competitive and can't wait to kick a soccer ball or throw basketballs into a hoop. The need to score obliterates any other awareness, sometimes resulting in knocking others over while focusing on scoring points. When another player interferes, the child might wail in anger. Competition tends to be one-sided for a young child.

The first two examples reflect children who need a slow

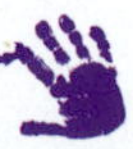

introduction to team participation. Careful assessment should be made regarding whether the time is ripe for a transition to a group setting or whether another season filled with smaller playdates might make the eventual transition to team play more successful. The fierce competitors might be ready for team play but require guidance in understanding the pros and cons of competition. Emphasis will need to be placed on learning to respect other team members and value other aspects of the game besides winning.

In his book *Child Development through Sports,* James H. Humphrey has identified specific social and emotional objectives that relate to participation in the sporting arena:[4]

- Children learn to work together.
- Children learn to accept and respect the rules of the game.
- Children learn to place the welfare of the group ahead of personal goals.
- Children learn to respect the rights of others.
- Team members think and plan as a group.
- Team members learn to win and lose gracefully.
- Sports provide fun and an emotional release.
- Children learn to control emotions, thereby facilitating emotional maturity.

Very young children generally are not that competitive, but competitiveness increases as children grow. There is a wide variety in the competitive edge among children, from very competitive to not competitive at all.[5] While it is the adults' responsibility to adjust the competition so it is a relatively even playing field, understanding how your child copes with competition is important.

There are many books that review indicators of a child's social and emotional readiness. These sources go into greater depth in assessing social interaction, separation issues, and emotional maturity. Similarly, many books have been written recently on the psychology of sports. Much has been discussed regarding the frame of mind of the athlete prior to and during a competition, which directly affects the athlete's performance. If the emotional readiness of a 250-lb defensive running back

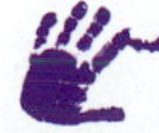

is key to his performance during a professional football game, imagine how pivotal it is for the 40-lb preschooler who's separated from the loving arms of Mommy for the first time.

Coaching and Instruction

Imagine this scenario. A team of third-grade boys battles for a victory on the soccer field. They lose, 3-2. As they begin to gather their belongings, the coach summons them to the bench for a lecture. The parents wait expectantly for 15 minutes. He proceeds to chew the boys out for not playing hard enough and then analyzes every bad play they made, criticizing almost every member of the team. Sadly, this is a true story.

Hopefully, this kind of "coaching" occurs infrequently. The National Youth Sports Coaches Association, or NYSCA, is a nonprofit organization that is a leader in the development of national training systems for volunteer coaches in youth sports. The objective is to help volunteer coaches understand the psychological, physical, and emotional effects they have on children aged 6-12 years old. NYSCA developed a Coach's Code of Ethics, including the rules and regulations coaches are required to observe. Little League Baseball, Inc, has provided similar information to their managers.[5]

These organizations help train and guide well-meaning adults in the ways of children. Understanding and appreciating the unique aspects of athletic growth in children as they move through various developmental phases is key to providing a supportive and healthy environment.

A University of California, Los Angeles, study of 2,000 children participating in sports showed that the number-one factor in enjoying the activity is having positive coach support. The lessons a good coach must impart are many. Coaches should consider the development of social awareness and social skills as important objectives. During game play, there are frequently emotionally charged situations. Not only should the coach help to diffuse the situation, but he or she should also use the crisis as an opportunity to teach children how to deal with strong emotions.[6]

Jordan Metzl, MD, discusses the coach-player relationship as potentially being very strong. The relationship gives the child

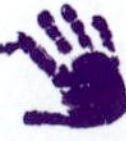

an opportunity to relate to another adult besides her parents. It is incumbent upon the coach to serve as a role model. The coach should consistently exhibit sportsmanship and fairness and value the whole child, not just how many goals the child scores.[7]

A Child's Expressed Interest and the Decision-Making Process

Most often, a child's expressed interest in a specific sport comes from familial, community, or cultural exposure.

Very few German children grow up without an interest in soccer. Soccer ("football") is played in the village park whenever the children are not in school and it is still light enough to see the ball. A 5-year-old will play in the same pickup game with the 12-year-olds. These are not adult-supervised sessions. They are juried by their peers. Team composition grows organically with the group that shows up that day. The size of the team expands and contracts as children come and go. The children's interest in the game may be fueled by the intense interest demonstrated by their family members, their community, and/or their country as a whole. Passion, coupled with patriotic pride, grips the entire nation as the World Cup games unfold.

In the U.S., sporting interests tend to vary. The feasibility of engaging in a specific sport should be considered. Availability, convenience, and cost are all realistic factors.

Consider the case of Max, a 6-year-old horse enthusiast. He always loved books about horses, had several play ponies, and decided he wanted to learn how to ride. While his mother Maria was able to pay for the 6-week introductory session offered by the local stable, the other accoutrements and long-term costs were prohibitive. She discussed this with her son, and they began to explore other sporting options.

Balancing the resources and needs of the family play an important part. If a child senses anxiety every time the family is packed into the car to drive 50 miles to the closest skating rink, the social and emotional implications may interfere with his enjoyment of the activity.

Once you determine as a family which sporting activities

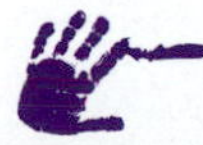

are feasible and available, your child's enthusiasm and interest should be the primary determinants of the ultimate choice.

Our achievement-oriented culture has created a myth that a child must start early and play often, if success is to be achieved in a sport. In essence, if a child does not begin serious participation in a formal sport as early as possible and with a high level of intensity, he will somehow miss his "window" to success.

Many star athletes' careers refute this assessment. Michael Jordan, the most gifted basketball player in recent history, didn't make the cut for the varsity team his sophomore year in high school and played junior-varsity basketball instead. Greg Norman, a celebrated professional golfer, has won 73 pro tournaments and is the third most lucrative player in golf history. He was born in Australia and spent his youth playing rugby and cricket. The first time he took up golf was at the age of 16, and within a year, he was a scratch golfer. Hakeem Olajuwon, a Nigerian soccer player, began playing basketball at the age of 17. He came to the United States and played basketball in college. His quick and nimble soccer footwork laid a great foundation for playing basketball, which led to a stellar career in the NBA. He is considered one of the all-time great centers and was nicknamed "Hakeem the Dream."

Often, we look at icons such as Tiger Woods, who did indeed begin playing golf at an early age, and we come to the erroneous conclusion that starting earlier is better. On the basis of Tiger's story, it would be easy to conclude that one must begin playing sports at the age of 2. The unwritten part of the story, however, is this: How many children began playing at an early age and quit? Or, how many children started early, yet played at an average to slightly above-average level throughout their lives? Research is missing on this point.

Contrast this against the situation in baseball in America today. There are currently more American children participating in Little League than ever. In spite of this, a large proportion of professional baseball "stars" come from a smattering of small communities in other countries that have few structured sports programs. Most of these players never joined a formal team until they were much older, often when scouts picked them out

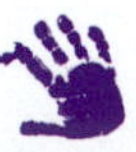

and plunked them into farm teams or Major League training teams. Most of their training came from casual but intense competition in their village pickup games, much the same way German children begin playing soccer.

The pressure to push a child into "elite" teams is tempting, especially as it can be an esteem builder for the child and often for the family. Keep in mind that highly talented athletes—those with superior motor-planning abilities—tend to rise to the top, no matter how and when they are introduced to a sport.

Just as parents need to assess when their child is ready to enter a sport, they need to go through a similar process when it comes to taking the activity to the next level. First and foremost, get a sense of whether your child loves the activity and wants to "eat, sleep, and breathe" it. Discuss with your child and coach whether there is enough challenge in the current venue or if your child needs to be playing with a more demanding group. Remember, some children learn to walk at 11 months, while others start at 14 months. By the time children enter preschool, no one is able to ascertain who is the better walker. The later walker will walk just as competently as the early walker.

Another star basketball player, Scottie Pippen, was not recruited for college ball. He played as a walk-on at the University of Central Arkansas and subsisted on a stipend as the basketball team manager until he grew to 6 feet 7 inches. By that time, he had developed sufficiently to be considered for pro ball and was recruited by the Seattle SuperSonics and the Chicago Bulls. He joined Michael Jordan in helping the Bulls win six NBA championships.[8]

The reason I share these stories is to help you as a parent relax about making athletic choices. Parents feel great pressure to make the right decisions for their children every day. Choosing a sport for a child should be a fun and stress-free process. It is not cast in stone, and changes can be made along the way.

Whatever the decision, it should lead to many hours of joy as your child develops new motor skills and learns to become a team player or performer. As you watch and enjoy this process and see a sense of competence and mastery develop in your child, you will know you have made good choices.

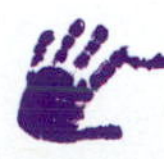

To review, the decision-making process includes the following considerations:

1. What activities are available?
2. Does the scheduling work?
3. Is the time commitment reasonable?
4. Is the activity affordable?
5. What is my child's interest level?

A note about discussing the available options with your child: It is important to *rule out activities that will not work* for your family *before* you present a list of choices to your child. Otherwise, your child may be disappointed and feel that the final decision you make as a family is a lesser choice. For example, if you do not have the time or resources to drive 60 miles out into the country twice a week for a horse-riding lesson, see if you can't come up with a more reasonable possibility that works for you and your family, instead. Presenting your child with a feasible alternative instead of an unrealistic one will spare him or her a possible disappointment and possibly allow a new solution to come into focus.

Before signing up for a specific team, carefully assess the coaching style. Talking with the league coordinators and speaking directly with the coaches to ascertain their philosophies and approaches are important steps in the vetting process. Observe a practice to see the coaches' style in action.

Moving your child on to the next level of competition, such as travel and elite teams, should be thought out carefully. Balancing your child's comfort level, the need for more intense competition, time commitment and demands, and a recommendation from the coaching staff should all come into play. Talk to parents who have done it both ways—going from delayed entry and gradually moving their child up to more intense levels, as well as those who chose to move their children up the ladder rapidly. Weigh the pros and cons of both approaches. Remember, each new season, a new decision can be made.

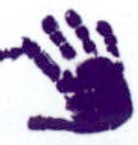

Playtime versus Structured Time

We've already reviewed the value of sports and the lessons imparted in a well-run program. During structured activities, your child learns lessons in sportsmanship, competition, specific skills, the value of hard work, and developing a sense of identity with a group or team. When your child engages in free play, many of these values come into play, but the dynamic shifts. Coached sports offer opportunities for the supervising adults to mediate and then teach lessons regarding sportsmanship and fair play. Unsupervised free play requires your young participant to make ongoing existential choices related to fairness and honesty. Strong opinions and varying approaches to competition play out in their "raw" form. The children must act "by the seat of their pants" in solving some of the conflicts that occur. Alliances build and break apart. Unkind acts, such as name-calling and an occasional punch, may occur.

The tendency of adults in recent times is to ward off and protect children from these hurtful infractions. The current method to do this is to set up highly structured environments where specific adults are sanctioned to be the authority figures. Children defer to the adults to manage them and make all the decisions. While this safeguards the children, it eliminates any opportunity for a child to assume a larger role in developing autonomous behavior and integrity.

During unsupervised play, it is important that children recognize that there are adults somewhere in the vicinity to rescue them if things spiral out of control at a level they cannot manage. This is why concepts such as those presented in *It Takes a Village*, by Hillary Clinton, are so important.[9] When adults take responsibility for all the children in the neighborhood, and respectful acceptance of positive and negative feedback occurs, children recognize that they are accountable not only to their own parents, but to others, as well.

In the 1950s, if Johnny was found smoking a cigarette behind the Jones's garage, you can bet Mrs Jones called Johnny's parents, and by dinnertime, Johnny was getting an earful. Today, there is a tendency to respect the privacy and the personal values of other families, which leads to a

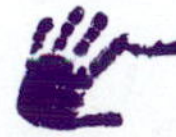

reluctance to interfere, even when you as an adult may have observed a behavior that is hurtful to your child or to others. Often "reporting" the observed behavior is not well received; in fact, frequently, the other child's family members become defensive and chastise a well-intentioned adult for accusing their child of wrongdoing.

Therefore, at the present time, children are left with two scenarios: *(a)* highly structured adult-driven activities and *(b)* completely unsupervised play. Of course, conscientious adults will frequently choose the seemingly "safer" choice of close adult supervision.

The trade-offs of shuttling your child from one activity to another should be weighed very carefully. In *The Hurried Child,* David Elkind reports that the hectic schedules we maintain today are turning our children into stressed, overwrought human beings.[10] In his book *Last Child in the Woods,* Richard Louv coins the phrase "nature-deficit disorder" and discusses the disadvantages of omitting nature exploration from the childhood experience.[11] The importance of unstructured free play during childhood is stressed by both authors.

As technology improves, neuroscientists continue to find growing evidence of the critical role that play has in forming and organizing developing young brains. Studies demonstrate how important movement and play are to cognitive and emotional development. In the building of neurological pathways, which are critical to being able to think and perform efficiently, rich and varied sensorimotor experiences are key in laying down the foundations for these "neurological superhighways."

While direct causal relationships have not been established between a lack of movement and/or unstructured play and attention-deficit disorder and other emotional and behavioral issues, trends indicate that as playtime shrinks, the number of diagnosed cases of behavioral disorders increases. The number of children participating in organized team sports is at an all-time high, yet Ritalin and other psychotropic medications are doled out in elementary schools at an alarming rate.

Similarly, the number of obese children in America is skyrocketing. Most children on the playing fields are not overweight, and one can argue that, thankfully, participation

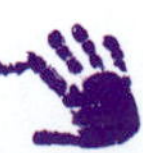

in structured sports single-handedly combats this scary trend. However, not all children participate in structured sports, sometimes for economic reasons, sometimes owing to problems with accessibility, and sometimes because the child is not fit enough or coordinated enough to join. It could even involve a simple a lack of interest. The culture of American childhood at present, however, does not provide a secondary, alternative outlet for healthy motor play. The child who is not ferried from one field to the next stays inside—and guess what? Turning on the computer or watching TV becomes the preferred activity.

Rethinking free time for children means stepping slightly outside the box. Free time provides opportunities that structured, adult-driven play will never provide. Unstructured playtime remains essential to healthy development. Understand that time without a plan is not wasted time. To paraphrase a popular credit card commercial, "Time to wander aimlessly and engage in whatever imaginary activity pops into the head at any given time…priceless!"

Childhood lasts a very short period of time in the human life span. It is the only time when a myriad of responsibilities does not fill most waking hours. How unkind is it to take the luxury of that time away from our boys and girls? While your weekly schedule is still in formation, think long and hard about the "enrichment" activities you allow time for in your child's life. Perhaps you could reassign which activities qualify as "enrichment." Just maybe, free time should head up the list.

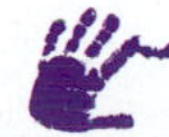

Notes

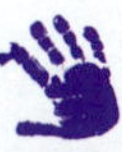

Chapter 7

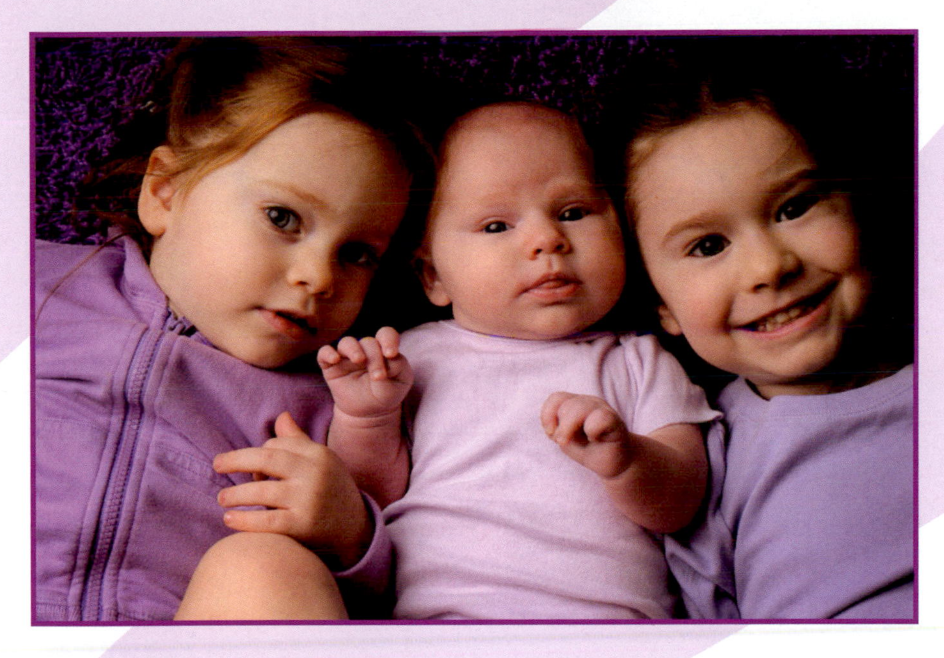

An Expanding View of Motor Skills

I still remember being a child and standing on the ledge of a rock stairway, deciding whether I should jump off. I weighed thoughts of a broken arm or leg realistically against my growing physical prowess. I had already broken a leg once before (screaming around a bend on a bicycle at 4 years old), so I understood the risks. I don't remember whether I jumped, but I do remember going through the decision-making process. When a child has an opportunity to make such a determination independently, the consequences are memorable. If the result is a trip to the emergency room with a broken arm, then the next time the child is confronted with a risk-taking experience, chances are, a more prudent decision will be made.

Earlier in this book, we focused on specific components of motor skills and the activities related to them. We talked about the importance of positioning to strengthen the trunk, engaging in activities to establish flexible movement patterns, and developing bilateral control, balance, and motor sequencing in various ways, as relates to a child's motor development. We've gone through specific motor activities and issues related to participation in sports and touched on the fact that a gifted or talented athlete will shine no matter what the circumstances, given ample opportunities to move around in the world in a healthy way.

We have not yet specifically discussed *how* one emerges as a talented athlete. So let's look at certain aspects in a child's makeup that help unravel the mystery of how some people become star athletes, how some manage to be middle-of-the-road performers, and how some come off as being genuinely klutzy. Physiology and body structure are obvious factors. No matter how beautiful the dancer, if the foot doesn't have a high arch, a career as a prima ballerina will not happen. Another critical factor, which is less understood, is the importance of motor-planning ability. Taking risks and making good decisions also play an important part.

Motor Planning

Imagine an adult tennis clinic. The tennis pro demonstrates a new technique to increase the speed of the ball when serving it. One student listens, observes the demonstration, and then

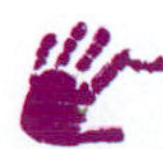

executes a perfect rendition of the intended action on the first try. Two more students try a few times, with mediocre success. The instructor may give more verbal cues, another demonstration, or even a few physical prompts to help them assimilate the new motor plan. After several more attempts, a slight increase in speed and effectiveness is seen—enough for the pro to say that the skill will solidify with practice. Then there is the fourth student, who attempts the new method of serving with disastrous results. The instructor provides all the same cues that were provided to the others, even adding additional instruction in an attempt to help this individual figure out how to execute the movement, to no avail.

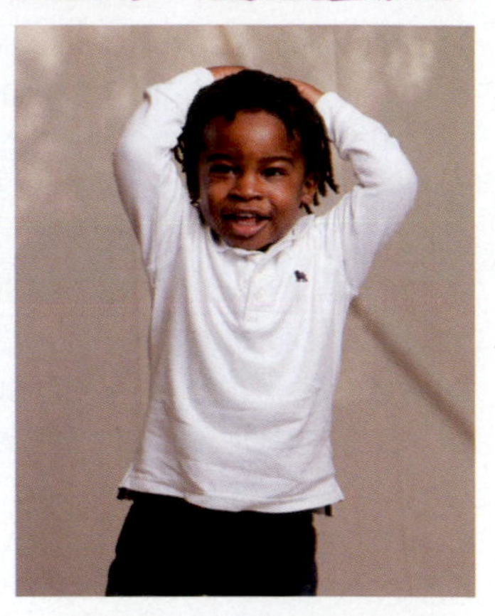

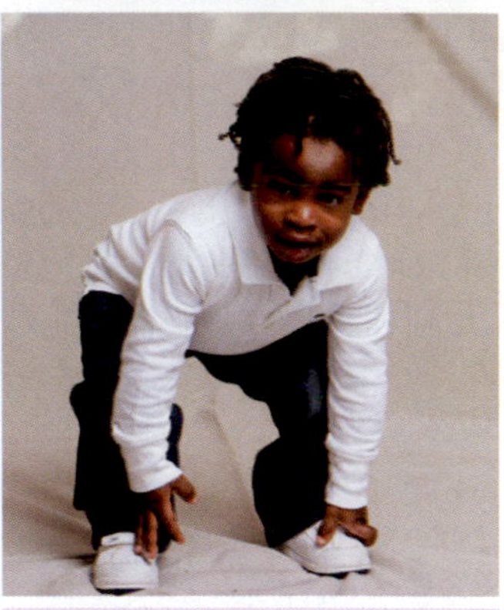

Figure 80. (a) and **(b)** Games to build body awareness. Here, Wayne plays "Head and Shoulders, Knees, and Toes."

The first student illustrates an example of *superior* motor-planning ability. This individual immediately grasps the concept or idea that the pro is attempting to impart. With a solid understanding of how the body works and feels, a strong and flexible body, well-coordinated use of both arms, good isolated control of body parts, and the ability to follow a motor sequence, this student executes with precision the first time. The fourth student is an example of someone with *motor-planning challenges*. Figuring out the concept or idea of the motor act may be the first roadblock. Fitness and strength may or may not be an issue, but the ability to coordinate the upper-body movements with the lower, the right side with the left, linking the necessary motor sequence together and integrating this with good eye-hand coordination becomes an insurmountable task.

Let's take this opportunity to talk more in-depth about motor planning. While a somewhat elusive concept, motor planning lurks and weaves its way around all motor actions, influencing

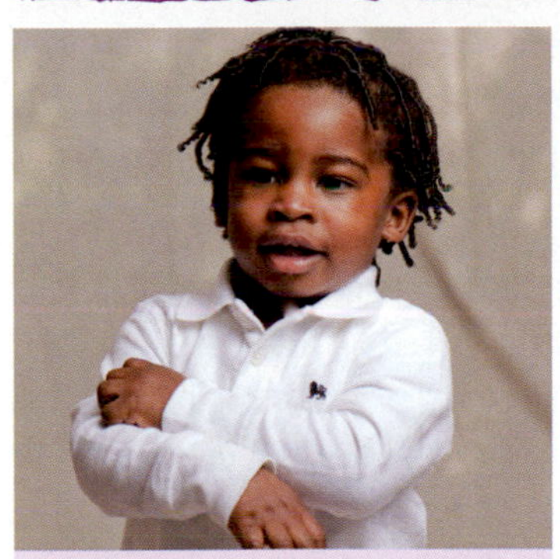

Figure 81. When playing body-awareness games, remember to add different body parts into the mix to increase your child's ability to discriminate his ankles from his hips, etcetera. Mix it up, as this helps keep your child flexible. Here, Wayne touches his elbows!

the quality, control, and ultimately the enjoyment of motor engagement. Motor planning is the official "glue" that allows some individuals to move rapidly to the front of the pack. Without this "glue," motor skills tend to fall apart. Participating in physical activities can be a frustrating and overwhelming challenge.

We've already mentioned several aspects of motor planning—body awareness, motor sequencing, and grading of movement all contribute to this complex and all-important process, which ultimately determines the athleticism of an individual. *Motor planning,* or *praxis,* is the ability to automatically figure out how to organize and execute a motor response. It relates not to the honing of a specific skill, such as batting a ball, but rather to the automatic and spontaneous ability to figure out *how to engage* in motor activity **(Figures 80 and 81)**.

Now imagine Tommy, a little boy who arrives at a new playground, immediately running up to the play structure and experimenting with ways to climb, jump, and swing. Another child, Sarah, needs encouragement and some instruction on how to proceed. Then there is Tad, who rushes headlong up a ramp, not accounting for the unfamiliar movement it entails, which results in a fall. Tad then charges over to another part of the play area. Rather than running around the sandbox, Tad trips over the edge. When Ellie arrives, she does not move toward the structure. Instead, she clutches her babysitter's leg. With some cajoling, Ellie eventually approaches the play structure but still clings to her sitter.

Tommy has established confidence in how his body moves and has acquired a general idea about how playgrounds work and how to proceed. With good body awareness and balancing, Tommy can make rapid adjustments to any sudden and unanticipated shifts in the structure. Developing motor skills allow him to explore different ways to play without receiving

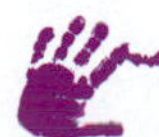

instruction from an adult. Tommy has strong motor planning. There is an inherent sense of confidence in how to approach and move his body while tackling the equipment. The playground is perceived as a thoroughly fun challenge.

Sarah needs some encouragement and moves toward the structure in a tentative way. She makes a realistic assessment of whether her body is ready for the unfamiliar demands of the equipment. Sarah's first steps on an unstable surface are slow and deliberate. Some trial-and-error movements occur as she figures out how to move safely.

Sarah's performance is typical of a child with average motor-planning abilities. The demands of the unfamiliar equipment are surmountable, but care and practice are required. After a certain amount of time, her confidence builds, and she enjoys exploring the new playground challenges. Most children fall into this category, reflecting typical and healthy motor development.

Tad is oblivious to the idea that there might be unforeseen challenges. His body is not equipped to adjust automatically to the new demands of the playground area. Sensing a shift in movement, which requires a specific body response, does not occur, leading to the resultant crash. Tad may become fearful from his fall, or he may be oblivious to it. Running headlong and tripping over the sandbox results from a lack of visual attention and spatial awareness of how to move around an object blocking his way. The effort required to plan and execute a shift in direction may be too much of a hassle. So, Tad runs toward it with the misguided idea that this is the path of least resistance.

Ellie lacks any confidence in how her body moves. She is fearful of the unstable walkway and doesn't know how to proceed. Ellie does not trust that her body will do what is required to negotiate the play structure successfully. She requires support and assurance that someone will be there to protect her in case of a misstep.

Motor planning has three basic components. The first relates to *ideation,* or the idea of how to approach a given motor task. The second relates to the ability to *link movements in the proper sequence and execute specific movements simultaneously*. The third relates to the *quality of actual execution*.

Ideation stems from an implicit understanding of how the body moves and responds in given situations. A good "motor memory" leads to moving in specific ways to execute motor tasks. Skill sets can be employed and redeployed in new configurations. These are automatically combined to form a plan for executing new motor activities. When previous responses do not quite fit the new situation, a new motor plan is generated automatically. At the same time, the brain has gathered all relevant information regarding the surroundings to execute this "plan" accurately. Amazingly, all of this occurs in a split second.

Then there is the case of Charlie, who struggled with the motor tasks of pumping and swinging. As he entered adolescence, he was determined to hone his basketball skills. Charlie practiced layups in the gym hundreds of times. He worked on the "dribble, step, shoot" sequence over and over again. He did it with precision, and eventually with ease. Charlie arrived at his neighborhood park, eager to show off his new skills. Sadly, having to dodge the opponents on the opposite team messed up Charlie's practiced pattern. While his heart was in it, he did not have the postural strength and body awareness required to rapidly alter his course of action. Charlie missed every shot and was relegated to being a second-string benchwarmer.

Contrast this against my son's friend, Pete, who joined us at the driving range one summer. This 10-year-old had never held a golf club before. However, Pete had been playing hockey throughout grade school. Physically fit, Pete had excellent eye-hand coordination from practicing hockey and related activities, coupled with having strong motor-planning ability. After a few demonstrations, Pete was driving the golf ball between 100 and 200 yards with every shot!

Once an idea is formed, the actual execution of the plan must occur. This is when all those motor components addressed earlier come together. Balance, coordinated use of both sides of the body, flexibility, rotation of the trunk, and sequencing of movement all play a part in how well a motor action occurs. Many motor-rich experiences throughout life help pull all of these components together.

The families I work with are wonderfully committed to helping their children grow. When activities are suggested to help work

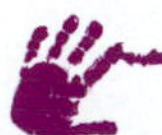

on specific sensorimotor areas, most parents diligently engage their child in whatever play activity has been recommended.

Jenny struggled with eye-hand coordination. She played catch with her dad every night when he came home from work. In spite of his patience and perseverance, Jenny persisted in throwing underhand, and when she attempted to reach over her head, the ball plopped to the ground several feet in front of her. This was not exactly the length needed to get the ball from home plate to first base. Jenny had not developed the trunk strength and flexibility to be able to reach spontaneously across her body as her right hand threw the ball. Her left arm stayed passively at her side. Her dad recognized the problem and helped her correct each component, but when she tried to put it all together, the ball simply landed at her feet. Besides lacking the foundations for good motor control, Jenny had difficulty combining several motor actions simultaneously and in sequence. These must be in place to be able to execute the action accurately and subsequently develop good motor planning.

On the other hand, Jenny's 3-year-old brother, David, watched these playtimes and retrieved the ball on occasion. While he was too young to have the upper-extremity strength and postural control to throw the ball very far, he automatically integrated the concept of throwing the ball overhead and crossing the midline of his body to follow through with the ball. He used his nondominant hand to help stabilize his trunk so he wouldn't fall. I mention David's abilities to illustrate the innate ability some lucky people have in figuring out, planning, and linking movements in a coordinated way from an early age. Jenny's dad will most likely be playing catch with David every night. He won't be teaching him to throw; rather, he will provide David with the athletic challenge David's little body demands.

As David and Jenny illustrate, motor planning ability *follows a continuum*. Where an individual falls on the spectrum depends in part on the genes dealt out at the time of inception. Whether these are fully expressed is dependent upon *environmental activation*. Put another way, having the potential to be a good athlete is part of the formula. The other part is *having the opportunity* to engage in many motor activities *early in and throughout childhood*. Just as intelligence is no longer considered a static factor, but rather a complicated process that integrates innate ability with experience, a child's motor-planning ability requires varied motor experiences to be able to reach his or her full potential.

Many of the children I have worked with had various motor weaknesses. As these areas improve, outstanding motor-planning ability frequently unfolds. A parent recently reported that her son, Paul, was becoming one of the top pitchers on his fifth-grade baseball team. When I worked with Paul, back in the second grade, he had poor muscle tone and some other issues primarily related to physical stamina. I had told his mother that in spite of his weak areas, he actually had excellent eye-hand coordination. Paul's mother confessed that she thought I was just trying to be nice and make her feel better about her son's limited motor ability. She was thrilled (and surprised) that my prediction came to fruition. I had stopped working with Paul when he was 7 years old. His mom and dad continued playing with him and engaging him in many physical activities—and it made all the difference.

Now let's turn to someone who clearly has the complete "gifted athlete" profile—Michael Phelps, the star swimmer of the 2008 Olympic games. While Michael Phelps's champion swimming record made his rise to stardom seem unsurprising, his road to athletic dominance was not always so clear-cut.

The winner of eight gold medals, Michael Phelps offers us an object lesson in someone who exemplifies the best of both biological and environmental conditions, which leads to attaining world-champion status. His mother, Deborah Phelps, relayed in an article, "He never sat still. He never shut up; he would never stop asking questions…he just wanted to go from one thing to another."[12] While school personnel worked with his family on managing Michael's attention-deficit disorder, Mrs Phelps signed her 9-year-old up for the swim club his older sisters belonged to. Fortunately for Michael, the coach, Bob Bowman, recognized unique potential in him. Even though he was still growing, Coach Bowman identified a physique that was perfectly matched to be a swimmer. He managed to work with Michael's hyperactivity and tolerated his behavioral transgressions. He imparted a work ethic and a sense of values in Michael, emphasizing not only hard work, but the importance of sportsmanship, as well. As a gifted coach, Bob was able to take the raw material he was presented with and develop Michael into a champion.[12]

Over time, Michael's body continued to develop. As Coach Bowman put it, Michael's "remarkably long torso is like the hull of a boat...allowing him to ride high in the water." Michael is extremely flexible, with a wingspan 3 inches longer than his 6-foot 4-inch height, and a size-14 foot. In addition, his body is able to recover faster than most, a phenomenon related to his personal level of oxygen consumption and uptake.[12]

Beyond his anatomy, physiology, and personality, Michael had a number of things going for him. His mother had the wisdom to recognize that this very active child was not a bad boy. He simply needed a physical outlet in which to channel his energy. As Mrs Phelps recounts, for the first 9 years of his life, Michael moved constantly, undoubtedly testing his physical limits on a regular basis. "Michael used to run around like a little crazy person...if he wasn't zooming by on his big-wheel tricycle, he was swinging past on the monkey bars."[13] She was fortunate enough to have the resources to place him in a good swimming program ("good" meaning that the program was a good fit for Michael—not that it trained nationally ranked athletes). Michael became engaged in the sport and learned to love swimming, and his coaches worked with his "raw materials" effectively. Of primary importance was the fact that Michael had a coach who understood physical development as well as the sport itself, so he knew when the time was ripe for Michael to commit in an intense way.

Undoubtedly, there were many other excellent swimmers in Michael's club. They did not, however, have all the stars lined up as Michael did. Committing to a rigorous swim program was the right thing for Michael to do. Few of us, however, have the ultimate combination of a perfect physique, the right physiology and mindset, and the innate motor ability to rise to a nationally ranked or professional level of a sport. For most of us mere mortals, motor planning and physical fitness develop through a variety of motor experiences. Some athletic abilities develop through practiced skill training, but many emerge through life experiences, especially in the realm of free play.

Note that Michael Phelps did not begin swimming seriously

until his 10th year. Before that, his mother described him as constantly in motion in noninstructional play. Playtime and free exploration, especially outside, allow a child to experiment with developing motor abilities, determine physical limits, and challenge himself to move beyond them.

Historical and Contemporary Perspectives of Play

For much of the 20th century, childhood was a time of meandering, with lazy days of self-exploration. A child had the time to explore the world independently. Children with an innate drive to engage in athletic endeavors had ample opportunities to run, roll down hills, climb trees, organize pickup games with flexible rules, and compete in the spirit of friendship. This was usually done in the exclusivity of peers, with no adults standing on the sidelines, cheering and evaluating.

The less athletically inclined children may have roamed the fields or woods, looking for interesting leaves and insects or catching frogs. This still required walking, bending over, reaching, and balancing when traversing over uneven surfaces, such as bogs, mud, and rocks. In the city, there was jumping rope, climbing walls, balancing on curbs, playing hopscotch, and organizing games of stickball in empty lots and alleys.

Childhood has always reflected the values of a culture at any given time. In America's infancy, the strict religious mindset highly influenced the raising of children. Adults viewed children as inferior beings that needed to be trained and turned into God-fearing adults. During the 18th and early 19th centuries, children were expected to assume adult roles at an early age. In their formative years, however, children were still allowed time to play. Parents were busy tending fields, doing household chores, and learning their trades. Entertaining one's children was not considered a parental obligation. Children were expected to entertain themselves. During the 1800s and early 1900s, values shifted considerably, and children were seen as unique entities who needed nurturing, along with the proper cultivation of values.[14]

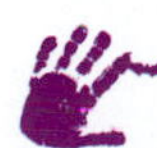

The 20th century brought incredible technological advancement and, with it, adults were freed up to pursue new interests. As the automatic washing machine became popular, women no longer slaved away at the washboard. Dishwashers, ready-made foods, take-out, and one-stop shopping all eased the burden of the homemaker. As the amount of leisure time increased, attention paid to the child intensified. In addition, television and other forms of media became a constant presence and began to influence most families' lives.

In *The Power of Play,* David Elkind describes hyperparenting, or what he calls a "helicopter parent," as a parent who hovers over everything a child does.[15] He explains that before World War II, parents were concerned about protecting a child's innocence. They were less concerned about protecting a child's physical well-being. "Parents allowed us to take risks and assumed that this is how we learned to deal with the real world. We got scrapes, bruises, and the occasional black eye, but that was part of growing up and learning to look after yourself."[16] As parents have lost more and more control over the information children are exposed to in today's media-driven world, childhood innocence is lost much earlier. Elkind suggests that "anxiety [related to] overprotecting our children's physical well-being may in part, at least, be a compensation for our relative inability to protect their psychological innocence...[as] we have lost control of the information flow to our children."

In other words, helicopter parenting may result from compensation due to feeling overwhelmed by our media-driven society and its interference. Or, parents may have too much time to devote to a child's every whim. In this litigious culture, a fear of lawsuits due to injury also contributes. Marketing forces have attempted to convince families that buying toys and programs leads to childhood enrichment and excelling in life. For whatever reason, it is clear that children spend significantly fewer hours in free unsupervised play these days than they do in outdoor play and unstructured play.

In his book about the loss of nature exploration and outside playtime, Richard Louv describes a culture that limits children's access to the outdoor world. He sites numerous studies that actually quantify the decreased amount of time children spend playing outside.[16] Studies on the comparison of two generations show a huge gap in the amount of time spent outdoors. Rhonda L. Clements's study showed that 71% of mothers reported playing outside every day as children, while 26% of their own children play outside daily today.[17] A study from the University of Glasgow showed that today's toddlers spend an average 20 minutes a day in physical activity.[18]

Playgrounds and parks offer opportunities for imaginative play and physical challenges unlike those found in a school gym or a family playroom. Crawling under bushes, climbing up on uneven rocks, and hiding in nooks and crannies all challenge the motor system in new and exciting ways. A child has to evaluate whether a jump from a rock 6 feet high might be too dangerous. These dynamic motor experiences lead to more flexible motor planning later in life. Risk assessment also improves.

Jane Clark, professor of kinesiology at the University of Maryland, talks about "containerized kids." Children spend a large portion of their day in car seats, high chairs, and strollers. As they get older, containerized experiences segue into sedentary screen-viewing experiences.[19] A 1998 National Survey showed that the average number of hours of television viewing per year was 1,500, compared with 900 hours of school.[20] How many hours of outdoor playtime would they have found if they had even asked? More recently, the trend has not changed for the better. A 2002 report showed that children 2 to 17 years old spend approximately 4.5 hours per day in front of some kind of screen. Two-and-a-half hours to 2.75 hours of that time is spent watching television.[21] With the digital explosion of MP3 players, smart phones, instant messaging, texting, tweeting, and all the other electronic gadgetry invented since 2002, imagine what the numbers are like this year!

While many parents talk about and understand the "evils" of television, the media, and computer games, few adults have questioned the intense overscheduling that has befallen our youth. While seemingly less alarming, parents frequently "manage" and overschedule their children. Usually this is done with the most sincere intent of enriching their children's lives. As a result, many children's afternoons (and evenings!) are dominated by Little League, soccer, dance, music, hockey, riding, pee-wee football, martial arts, lacrosse, basketball, swimming, tennis, golf, drama, chess, nature classes, science and math enrichment, tutoring, scouts...and the list goes on.

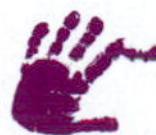

All of these activities provide valuable experiences, but they are *adult driven*. The child is not primarily responsible for the process. The opportunity for independent play and independent decision-making is taken away. The child's opportunities to develop autonomy and independence are diminished at best, and, for the completely overscheduled child, stripped away entirely. One needs to weigh the value of independent playtime against the advantages of these other activities. When Susie is signed up for classes from 2:30 to 6:00 every day, there is no time left for her to play.

Organized sports and other activities provide wonderful opportunities for children to socialize, learn about a particular activity, and begin the process of developing rudimentary skills in that specific activity. What they don't offer is unsupervised time in which a child must engage in decision-making and negotiation with peers without adult intervention. Free play occurs without the watchful eye of an adult, and, as such, a child can engage in silly and nonpurposeful activities that help him or her learn about the limits and abilities of the body that might not otherwise be tested. Unsupervised play and engagement in motor activity is assessment free.

David Elkind points out that the decrease in opportunities for children to engage in self-initiated games coincides with Americans losing preeminence in baseball, as was alluded to earlier. Despite the more than 3 million American children involved in Little League and numerous baseball camps, Caribbeans, Central Americans, and South Americans are increasingly becoming the stars of our professional teams. Many of these players grew up playing for the fun of it and never participated in organized teams, such as Little League.[22] While reaching national status in professional sporting teams may not be the goal of most parents, other values derived from unstructured play may be.

Play is the dominant form of learning for a child; therefore, eliminating unsupervised play deprives a child of self-created learning experiences. Overprotection has a profound effect on children's play. When children play on their own, there are many opportunities for innovation and invention. Children learn to relate to one another and resolve conflicts, even if this occasionally involves fights. Organized play robs a child of opportunities to learn from risk-taking behaviors.[22]

Brain Development through Motor Activity

About 2,300 years ago, Plato suggested that all early education should be a sort of play and should develop around play situations. The philosophers Locke and Rousseau both emphasized that learning should develop from enjoyable activities of childhood.[23] George Herbert Mead, the father of social psychology, states, "Children learn social responsibility, to relate to others, and to integrate themselves within the social collective." In playing a game, a child must be ready to handle the attitude of everyone involved in the game.[24]

These philosophers intuitively saw the value of play. New technology has borne out the importance of play and sensorimotor engagement in brain development. This includes learning, attention, and behavioral and emotional development. In her book *Failure to Connect,* Jane Healy discusses brain-development research that points to the key roles play and movement have in this process. Studies have shown that groups of rats living in enriched environments (with larger cages and more playmates, wheels, and balls) had significant increases in the size of their cortexes (the thinking part of the brain), more connections between synapses, and an increase in glial support cells and neurons, with more dendritic spines. This essentially means that when the rats lived in more enriched environments, their brains subsequently became more highly developed, with better organization and communication of information. What constituted an "enriched environment?" One that provided active engagement in play, movement, socialization, and novelty.[25]

Healy points out that physical and social experiences are intricately tied to a young child's mental development.[25]

"For the young child, movement and physical experience provide the foundation for higher-level cognition through integration of the brain's sensory association areas. Certain visual-spatial skills that contribute to math and science thinking are also learned from using the whole body to navigate through space while running, jumping, climbing, etc. The child's muscles are 'smart instruments' that register the spatial properties of

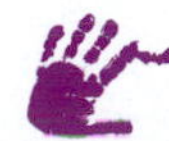

objects in the environment and build a foundation for higher conceptual understanding (proportion, velocity, engineering, [and] design)."[26]

The neuroanatomist Marian Diamond states, "Do not neglect the fact that the cortex does not work alone. Children need a multisensory, enriched environment...children need to run, hop, and jump and do all the other things that kids do to develop the whole (cortical) mantle."[27] Healy asks the question, "Who knows how much of the escalating degree of social and personal malaise present in today's young people is a function of too much electronic stimulation replacing physical activity and interpersonal experience?"[28]

A neurological process occurs throughout child development that helps the brain work more efficiently. One process is called "synaptic pruning." "During the early years, the (neurons) that get used are the ones that will be strengthening and survive. A major task of childhood is to prune this mass of potential into networks of connections that are useful and automatic for the mental skills that this particular child is encouraged to develop."[28] If pruning does not occur, Healy warns, the child's mind might resemble a "booming, buzzing confusion."

As we've talked about before, infants and toddlers need to spend most of their waking hours engaged in movement. Healy points out that the body experiences of this early age lead to planning, coordinating, and sequencing movements. She provides examples of hammering and throwing a ball, both of which require an exact sequence of activation of dozens of neurons and muscles.

Between 4 and 7 years of age, language guides motor actions and attention.

This leads to the ability to:[28]

- *Plan* and *sequence* specific tasks.
- *Learn* to switch activities.
- *Concentrate,* even if boring.
- *Complete tasks* independently.
- *Think* before acting impulsively or hurtfully.
- *Understand* others' feelings.

Current Trends in Play

The value of play in the late 20th and early 21st centuries has become a commercial commodity. Play frequently takes place in structured settings, such as team sports, mini gyms, and indoor play environments. *The Last Child in the Woods* author Richard Louv discusses the criminalization of unstructured natural play. He points out that countless communities have virtually outlawed unstructured outdoor natural play, often because of the threat of lawsuits but also increasingly due to a growing obsession with order.[29]

Along with "adult-only" communities, the tolerance for children playing outside in the community has diminished significantly. Carter Dougherty of *The New York Times* reported on litigation involving a childcare center in Hamburg, Germany. A neighbor filed a lawsuit about noise made by the children at the center. Complaints of noisy children have apparently become a frequent occurrence throughout Germany. Often, neighbors don't bother to speak with daycare centers or schools before calling the police. Some complaints are settled by limiting the times that the children spend outside. In the Hamburg case, while neighbors fretted over the noise level generated by the child center, the center was located directly across from bus and commuter train stations, along a busy thoroughfare, and directly in the approach of a landing strip for the Airbus, which lands approximately a dozen times a day. The cargo aircraft is described as resembling "beluga whales with thrusters roaring over the neighborhood at low altitudes."[30]

People have apparently assimilated mechanical noises better than the squeals of children's laughter. This phenomenon is not unique to Germany. A similar case occurred in the affluent community of Greenwich, Connecticut. The case involved a town-owned vacant lot, a few industrious teenage boys with a Kevin Costner–type vision of a "Field of Dreams," and "angry neighbors and a bevy of lawyers, police, and town officials," Peter Applebome, of *The New York Times,* writes.[31]

> After three weeks of clearing brush and poison ivy, scrounging up plywood and green paint, digging holes and pouring concrete, about a dozen teenagers built a version of Fenway Park, complete with a 12-foot-tall

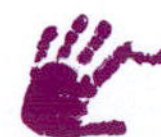

> green monster in center field [and an] American flag by the left field pole...it turns out that one kid's field of dreams is an adult's dangerous nuisance, liability nightmare, inappropriate usurpation of green space, unpermitted special use, or drag on property values. The Wiffleball Fenway has become...a suburban Rorschach test about youthful summers past and present.

And how did such attention come to be focused on the industrious endeavor of a few teenage boys unplugging their computers and working together on a constructive activity? The property owner behind the lot said, "If I come home at six at night after work all day, I want peace and quiet. I can't have that. I have dozens of people behind my house playing Wiffleball."[31]

Here is an object lesson on the quiet crisis confronting childhood in the 21st century. At a time when child specialists sound alarms about the overuse of electronics and the exclusion of wholesome outside play, this story highlights the complicating forces that diminish and compromise normal and healthy childhood practices. Lawsuits abound, leading to individuals refusing to share their property, such as a perfect sledding hill, because they fear potential lawsuits from an inadvertent injury occurring on the premises.

The thought of children engaging in an activity without adult control is anathema to today's highly scheduled and structured society. In the Greenwich case, a group of young teenagers chose to turn off their computers and electronic toys to get some fresh air and exercise and engage in a resourceful project that brought them together in a positive way. Rather than heralding this as an industrious and creative project, the grown-up regulatory powers-that-be came knocking. Certainly there may have been regulatory issues that required adult guidance. Instead of lending a helping hand, however, the bureaucratic machine stepped in and shut down the park. How many children in that town will attempt a similar creative endeavor in the future? When an affluent community chooses to censure wholesome play, it brings into question the overall health of childhood and the corresponding development of physical and neurological maturation.

While developing skills and competence in computers and

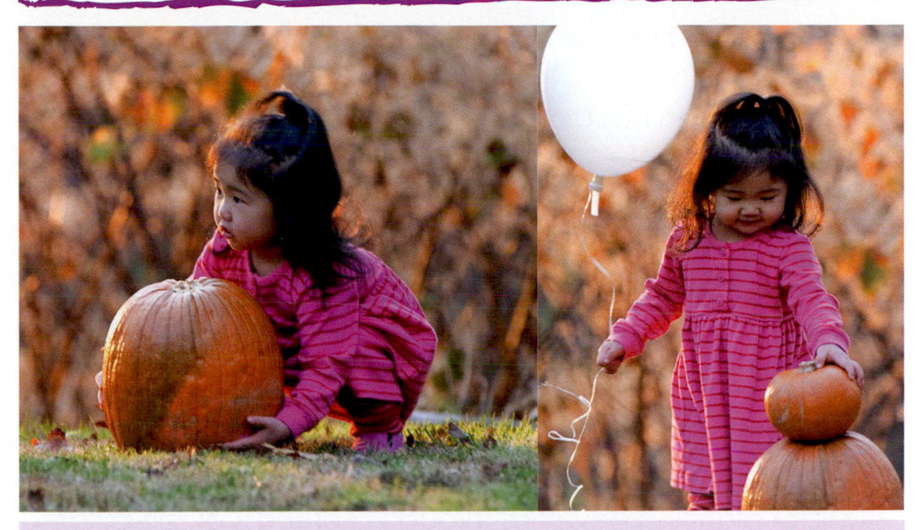

Figure 82. (a) Learning about the world from the natural environment is very important. Elisa will remember the concepts of "round" and "heavy" as she tries unsuccessfully to lift this pumpkin. **(b)** Voila! Small pumpkins can be lifted, balloons are big but light…and huge pumpkins make great bases for stacking.

other electronic-related activities is important at some time during the school years, we need to address what is lost in the hours spent staring at a screen.

To start with, concern should be raised on a physical level. Remember the discussion of dynamic balancing and how many adult exercise programs are incorporating this into their regimes because adults "have been sitting at their desks for years"? Are we creating children who "sit at their desks for years"? In the case of adults, returning to exercise regimes reactivates muscles that are long underused but had been strong years ago, in childhood. If children are spending hours upon hours in the backseat of a car (and at the most critical early years, tethered in the even more cramped quarters of a car seat) and then saddled up to a computer screen for the remainder of the day, think of the muscles that are not getting stronger. And think of the neural pathways that are not developing!

Consider the overall physical fitness of your child. Fast food is not the only culprit of rising childhood obesity levels. Think of the missed opportunities to explore nature and engage in social and imaginary play. What critical lessons in the physical world, which serve as a platform for basic conceptual thinking in math and science, do not get learned? What would Socrates

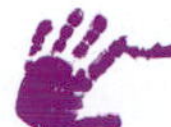

and Plato have to say about the current state of our children's upbringing?

The discussion has broadened beyond motor planning and the acquisition of motor skill development. Keep in mind the old adage, "We learn from doing." Our first life experiences relate to our senses and how we move in the world. Language develops and becomes a major player in a child's life experience. The need to keep moving is imperative, however. Exploring physical limits, providing the brain with valuable sensorimotor nutrition (or stimuli), and learning new ways to move and approach the world help a child become proficient in movement. Keeping active also helps develop flexible strategies in approaching and subsisting in the world around us.

Motor planning develops through a process of self-initiated motor learning. It begins with an infant's response to her mother's face, voice, and touch. Primitive reflexes segue into intentional movements. Opportunities to play at each level of development help cement a sense of self and develop competence in her ability to interact with her surroundings. Movement and the associated sensory input derived from motor activity help build efficient neural pathways, which are critical for concentration, organization of thought, and high-level conceptual learning. As a child grows, these opportunities need to expand, not contract. Athletic opportunities are one way to continue developing motor planning and physical ability. Random, unstructured play is another. It is critical that time is set aside each day for both to happen **(Figure 82)**.

Recommended Activities

- Engage your baby in a sensorimotor–rich environment at an early age. This includes many opportunities for movement, both passive and active. Incorporate a combination of tactile exploration and visual and auditory stimuli in each experience so your child learns to integrate stimuli from multiple sources automatically.
- Continue to engage your baby in novel movement activities. When your child is crawling on the floor, toss a pillow in his path to create a problem-solving scenario (how to get over or around it).
- Provide simple challenges for your toddler. Pile pillows and cushions on the floor for him to climb over. Leave a large cardboard box in the middle of the room so he can figure out how to turn it into a house or whatever his imagination creates.
- Remember that your child, from birth through his 8th year, remains in the sensorimotor phase of development. This means that motor or movement opportunities should occur throughout his waking hours. Sitting in a car does not provide adequate sensorimotor experiences, so time spent in the car should be gauged very carefully. The same goes for watching television and videos.
- Free play remains critical during the 3- to 8-year-old period. Children should have the opportunity to play without adult-directed intervention every day. As your child grows and your schedules get cramped, try to reassess your priorities if a large chunk of time per week is not devoted to free play.
- For a younger child, "unsupervised play" means an adult is at hand to make sure your child remains safe but does not direct the actual activity. Working in the kitchen, folding laundry, and working on the computer with a vigilant eye will teach your child that grown-ups have obligations independent of him or her, just as your child needs to develop play skills without requiring adult direction.

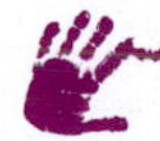

- Older children will benefit from play where adults are absent. Safety parameters should be established, such as where the child is allowed to go and for how long. Presumably, at this point, the child has learned basic safety and courtesy rules and regulations of the community.
- Structured activities, such as sports, can be a valuable and enjoyable part of a child's growing years. However, make sure that unstructured time is still a major component in your child's schedule. If the ratio is tipped in favor of structured activities, it may be time to reassess your priorities.

References

1. Greenspan S, Brazelton TB. *The Irreducible Needs of Children*. Cambridge, MA: De Capo Press; 2000.
2. Chopra D. Simon D, Abrams V. *Magical Beginnings, Enchanted Lives: A Holistic Guide to Pregnancy and Childbirth*. New York, NY: Three Rivers Press; 2005:257.
3. Humphrey JH. *Child Development through Sports*. New York, NY: The Hayworth Press; 2003:53.
4. Humphrey JH. *Child Development through Sports*. New York, NY: The Hayworth Press; 2003.
5. Humphrey JH. *Child Development through Sports*. New York, NY: The Hayworth Press; 2003:54,57.
6. Humphrey JH. *Child Development through Sports*. New York, NY: The Hayworth Press; 2003:57.
7. Metzl J. *The Young Athlete*. New York, NY: Little, Brown & Company; 2002.
8. Scottie Pippen. Wikipedia. http://en.wikipedia.org/wiki/Scottie_Pippen. Accessed March 22, 2011.
9. Clinton H. *It Takes a Village*. New York, NY: Simon & Schuster; 1996.
10. Elkind D. *The Hurried Child: Growing Up Too Fast Too Soon*. Cambridge, MA: Da Capo Press; 2001.
11. Louv R. *Last Child in the Woods*. Chapel Hill, NC: Algonquin Books of Chapel Hill; 2005.
12. Michaelis V. Built to swim, Phelps found a focus and refuge in water. *USA Today*. July 31, 2008.
13. Winerip M. Phelps's mother recalls helping her son find gold-medal focus. *New York Times*. August 8, 2008:W4.
14. Mintz S. *Huck's Raft, A History of American Childhood*. Cambridge, MA: The Belknap Press of Harvard University Press; 2004.
15. Elkind D. *The Power of Play*. Cambridge, MA: De CapoPress; 2007:76,79.
16. Louv R. *Last Child in the Woods*. Chapel Hill, NC: Algonquin

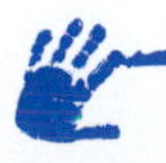

Books of Chapel Hill; 2005:10,34-36,100,159.

17. Clements R. An investigation of the state of outdoor play. *Contemp Issues Early Child.* 2004;5(I):68-80.
18. Reilly J, Jackson D, Montgomery C, et al. Total energy expenditure and physical activity in young Scottish children: mixed longitudinal study. *Lancet.* January 2004;363(9404):211-212.
19. Louv R. *Last Child in the Woods*. Chapel Hill, NC: Algonquin Books of Chapel Hill; 2005:35.
20. Oklahoma State University Web site. Cooperative Extension. Children and Families Parenting Issues. http://fcs.okstate.edu./parenting/. Accessed February 16, 2011.
21. Gentile DA, Walsh DA. *App Dev Psychol.* 2002;23:157-178.
22. Elkind D. *The Power of Play*. Cambridge, MA: De CapoPress; 2007:80-82.
23. Humphrey JH. *Child Development through Sports*. New York, NY: The Hayworth Press; 2003:50.
24. Elkind D. *The Power of Play*. Cambridge, MA: De CapoPress; 2007:149.
25. Healy J. *Failure to Connect*. New York, NY: Simon and Schuster; 1998:70-71,219-220.
26. Calvin WH. The emergence of intelligence. *Sci Am.* October 1994:101-107.
27. Diamond M. Computers and cognitive development. Invitational workshop presented at: University of California, Berkeley; November 17, 1996.
28. Healy J. *Failure to Connect*. New York, NY: Simon and Schuster; 1998:74,171.
29. Louv R. *Last Child in the Woods*. Chapel Hill, NC: Algonquin Books of Chapel Hill; 2005:27-34.
30. Dougherty C. Sturm und drang about pint-size neighbors. *New York Times.* January 28, 2009:A3.
31. Applebone P. Build a Wiffle ball field and lawyers will come. *New York Times*. July 10, 2008.

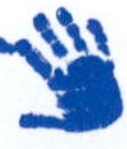

Recommended Reading

Touchpoints Birth to Three, by T. Berry Brazelton, MD. Cambridge, MA: De Capo Press, 2006.

Magical Beginnings, Enchanted Lives: A Holistic Guide to Pregnancy and Childbirth, by Deepak Chopra, MD, and David Simon, with Vicki Abrams. New York, NY: Three Rivers Press, 2005.

First Feelings, by Stanley Greenspan, MD, and Nancy T. Greenspan. New York, NY: Penguin Books, 1985.

The Happiest Baby on the Block, by Harvey Karp, MD. New York, NY: Bantam Dell, 2002.

Why Motor Skills Matter, by Tara Losquadro Liddle, MPT, with Laura Yorke. New York, NY: Contemporary Books, 2004.

The Baby Book, by William Sears, MD, and Martha Sears, RN. New York, NY: Little Brown and Company, 2003.

The Baby Bible, by Birgit Gebauer-Sesterhenn and Manfred Praun, MD. New York, NY: Barron's, 2005.

Your Baby and Child: From Birth to Age Five, by Penelope Leach. New York, NY: Dorling Kindersley Book of Random House, 1977.

Child Development through Sports, by James H. Humphrey. New York, NY: The Hayworth Press, 2003.

The Young Athlete, by Jordan D. Metzl, MD, with Carol Shookhoff. New York, NY: Little, Brown, and Company, 2002.

Raising a Sensory-Smart Child, by Lindsey Biel, MA, OTR/L, and Nancy Peske. New York, NY: Penguin Books, 2005.

The Hurried Child: Growing Up Too Fast Too Soon, by David Elkind. Cambridge, MA: Da Capo Press, 2001.

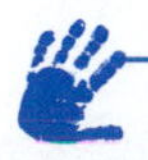

The Power of Play: Learning What Comes Naturally, by David Elkind. Philadelphia, PA: De CapoPress, 2007.

Failure to Connect, by Jane M. Healy, PhD. New York, NY: Touchstone Books, 1998.

Your Child's Growing Mind: Brain Development and Learning from Birth to Adolescence, by Jane M. Healy, PhD. New York, NY: Broadway Books, 1987.

Different Learners, by Jane M. Healy, PhD. New York, NY: Simon and Schuster, 2010.

The Out-of-Sync Child, by Carol Stock Kranowitz, MA. New York, NY: Perigee Books, 2005.

The Out-of-Sync Child Has Fun, by Carol Stock Kranowitz, MA. New York, NY: Perigee Books, 2006.

Raising an In-Sync Child, by Carol Stock Kranowitz, MA. New York, NY: Perigee Books, 2010.

The Last Child in the Woods, by Richard Louv. Chapel Hill, NC: Algonquin Books of Chapel Hill, 2008.

Huck's Raft: A History of American Childhood, by Steve Mintz. Cambridge, MA: The Belknap Press of Harvard University Press, 2004.

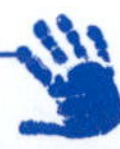

About the Author

Jill has worked with children for more than 30 years as an occupational therapist. Through her private practice of 25 years, she specializes in sensory integration and other developmental issues. Jill has helped families who struggle with a variety of special needs, ranging from autism to attention-deficit disorders. An early pioneer in sensory integration and Sensory Processing Disorder, Jill understood the impact of sensorimotor development on emotions and behaviors long before psychologists and the mainstream medical community caught on. Today, she continues to work with children and educators in a consultative role for both normally developing children and those with special needs. In addition, Jill gives talks to parent groups and educators on sensorimotor development.

After receiving her undergraduate degree from the University of Pennsylvania, Jill went on to complete a master's degree in counseling and human relations from Villanova University. She did her advanced graduate work, including a teaching fellowship, at New York University. She has served on many boards, including a term as co-president of Ridgefield, A Better Chance program, and is a founding member of the Connecticut Council for Vital Voices Global Partnership.

Her publications have been professional in nature. She has written articles regarding special education and miscellaneous topics in local newspapers. She has also developed promotional materials for the organizations with which she has been involved.

A mother of three, Jill adds 26 years of parenting to her professional experience with children.

This is Jill's first book, which she felt compelled to write after people who have attended her talks enthusiastically suggested she take on this challenging task. She continues to write about motor development on her Web site and blog, *www.TheMotorStory.com*.

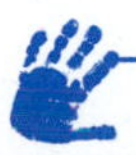

Additional Resources

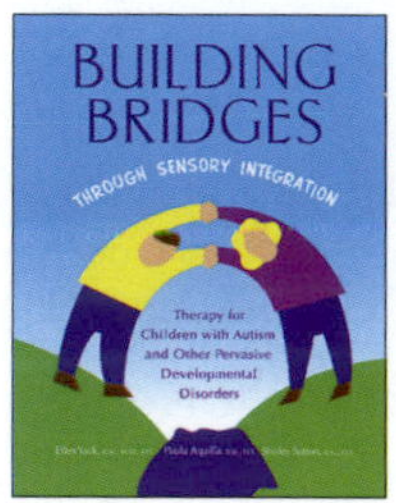

Paula Aquilla, Ellen Yack, & Shirley Sutton
Building Bridges through Sensory Integration, 2nd edition
www.sensoryworld.com

Britt Collins & Jackie Olson
Sensory Parenting: From Newborns to Toddlers—Everything Is Easier When Your Child's Senses Are Happy!
www.sensoryworld.com

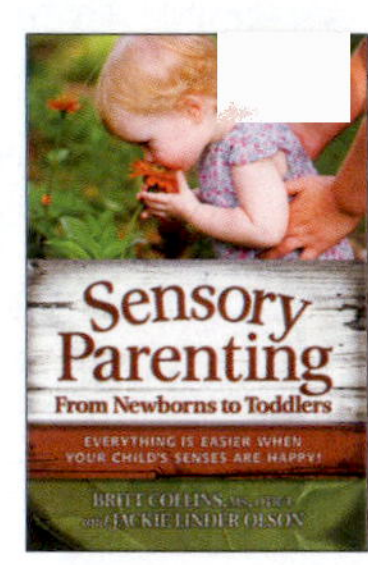

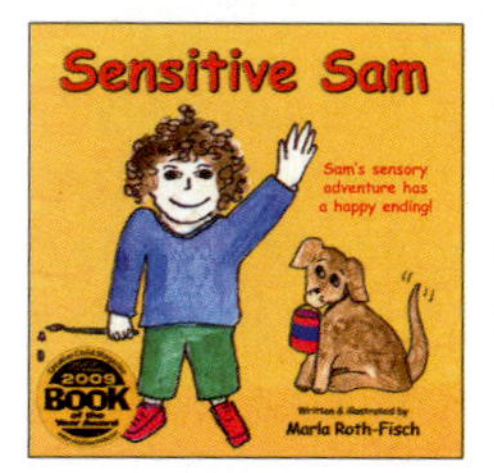

Marla Roth-Fisch
Sensitive Sam: Sam's sensory adventure has a happy ending
www.sensoryworld.com

Dr. Temple Grandin
The Way I See It and *Thinking in Pictures*
www.fhautism.com

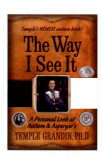

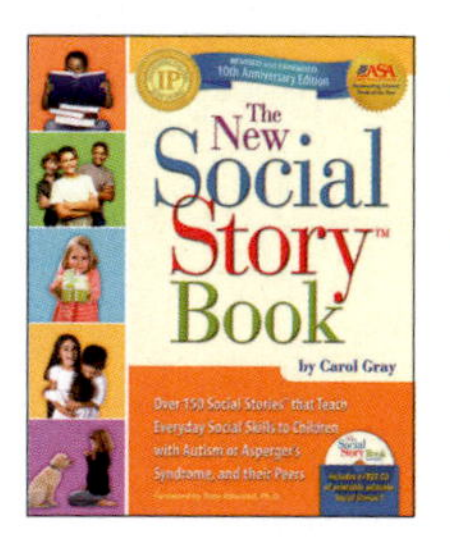

Carol Gray
The New Social Story Book
www.fhautism.com

Jennie Harding
Ellie Bean, the Drama Queen
www.sensoryworld.com

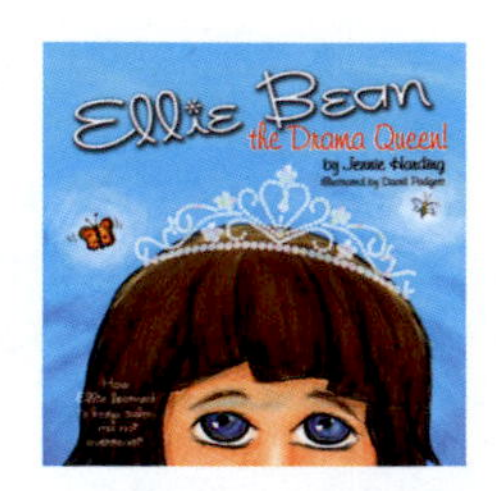

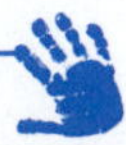

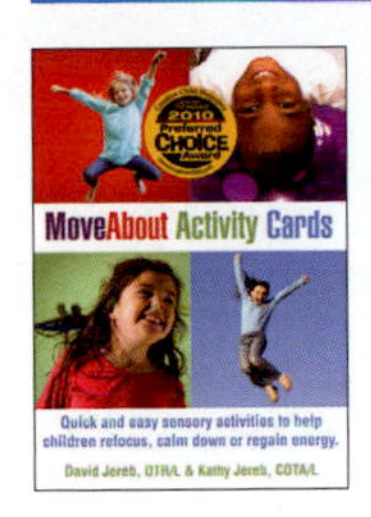

David Jereb & Kathy Koehler Jereb
MoveAbout Activity Cards: Quick and Easy Sensory Activities to Help Children Refocus, Calm Down or Regain Energy
www.sensoryworld.com

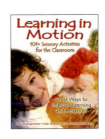

Joan Krzyzanowski, Patricia Angermeier, & Kristina Keller Moir
Learning in Motion: 101+ Fun Classroom Activities
www.sensoryworld.com

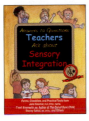

Jane Koomar, Stacey Szklut, Carol Kranowitz, et al
Answers to Questions Teachers Ask about Sensory Integration
www.sensoryworld.com

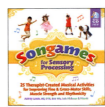

Aubrey Lande & Bob Wiz
Songames™ for Sensory Processing (CD)
www.sensoryworld.com

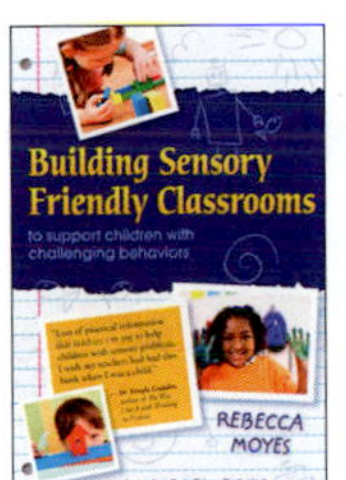

Rebecca Moyes
Building Sensory Friendly Classrooms to Support Children with Challenging Behaviors
www.sensoryworld.com

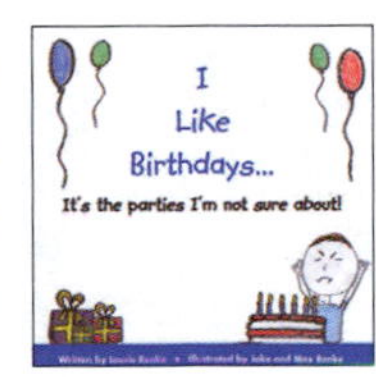

Laurie Renke, Jake Renke, & Max Renke
I Like Birthdays...It's the Parties I'm Not Sure About!
www.sensoryworld.com

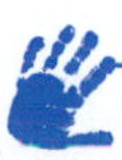

John Taylor, PhD
Learn to Have Fun with Your Senses!
The Sensory Avoider's Survival Guide
www.sensoryworld.com

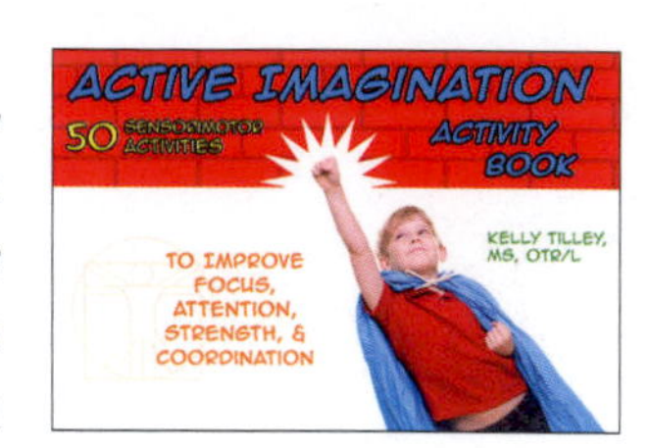

Kelly Tilley, MS, OTR/L
Active Imagination Activity Book:
50 Sensorimotor Activities to Improve
Focus, Attention, Strength, & Coordination
www.sensoryworld.com

Carol Kranowitz, MA
The Out-of-Sync Child, 2nd ed;
The Out-of-Sync Child Has Fun, 2nd ed;
Getting Kids in Sync (DVD featuring the children of St. Columba's Nursery School);
Growing an In-Sync Child;
Sensory Issues in Learning & Behavior (DVD);
The Goodenoughs Get in Sync;
Preschool Sensory Scan for Educators (Preschool SENSE) Manual and Forms Packet

www.sensoryworld.com

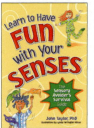

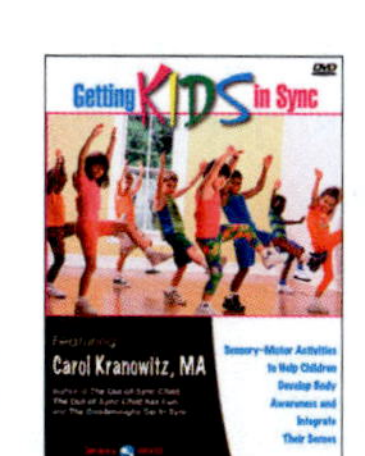

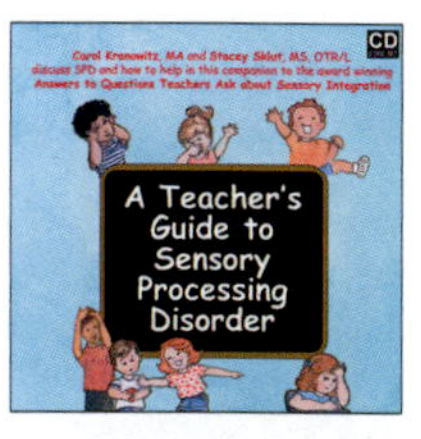

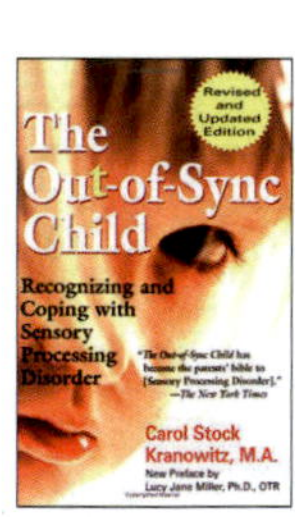

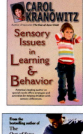

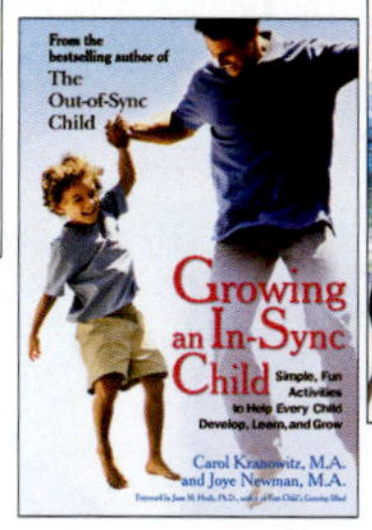

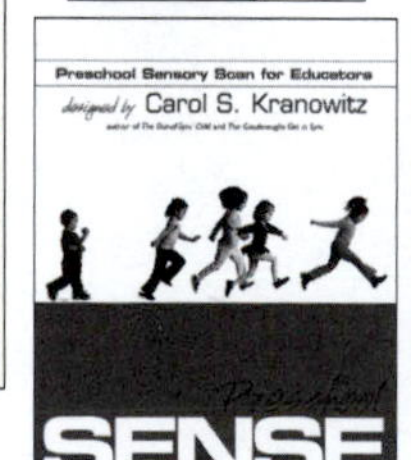

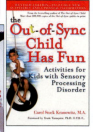

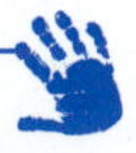

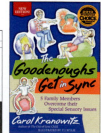

INDEX

A

B

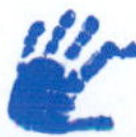

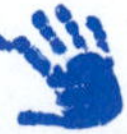

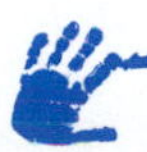

K

L

M

N

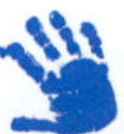

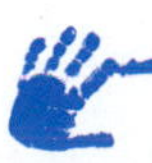

S

T

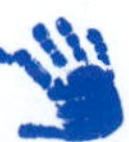

U

V

W

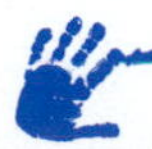

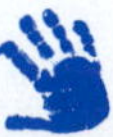